Contents

Prevention of disabilities in patients with leprosy

A PRACTICAL GUIDE

H. Srinivasan

former Director
Central JALMA Institute for Leprosy
Agra, India

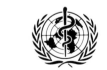

World Health Organization
Geneva
1993

WHO Library Cataloguing in Publication Data

Srinivasan, H.
    Prevention of disabilities in patients with leprosy : a practical guide.

    1.Leprosy – complications   2.Leprosy – therapy   I.Title

    ISBN 92 4 154456 2   (NLM Classification: WC 335)

TYPESET IN INDIA
PRINTED IN ENGLAND
92/9512 –Macmillan/Clays – 7000

Foreword

Leprosy continues to be of major concern in developing countries, not only because of the large numbers of people affected by it and their potential for communicating the disease to others, but also because of the occurrence of deformities in a proportion of patients. While the introduction and widespread application of multidrug therapy over the past decade has resulted in significant reductions in the incidence of the disease, the impact on the associated disabilities and deformities has been very limited. Action is needed in order to prevent, limit and correct deformities among individuals who have or have had the disease. It is in this context that this guide, outlining the measures and actions for disability prevention that need to be undertaken at field level, has been prepared.

The guide is based on the recommendations of a WHO Consultation on Disability Prevention and Rehabilitation in Leprosy, which met in Geneva from 9 to 11 March 1987. The manuscript and illustrations were prepared by Dr H. Srinivasan, whose contribution is gratefully acknowledged. Acknowledgement is also due to those who reviewed the manuscript and provided many useful suggestions and criticisms. The reviewers included: Dr P. Bourrel, formerly Professor at the Institute of Tropical Medicine, Marseille, France; Dr P. Brand, formerly of the Department of Health and Human Services, Gillis W. Long Hansen's Disease Centre, Carville, LA, USA; Dr F. Duerksen, Lauro de Souza Lima Hospital, Bauru, São Paulo, Brazil; Dr L. N. N'Deli, formerly of the Raoul Follereau Institute, Adzope, Côte d'Ivoire; and Dr D. D. Palande, formerly of the Sacred Heart Leprosy Centre, Sakkottai, Kumbakonam, India.

Even though this guide is not a formal training manual, it can still be used as a teaching aid. It does not address a specific category of health worker, since it is expected that the responsibility for disability prevention will vary in different countries and in different areas in a country. Because of the diversity of the audience, only a very limited amount of theoretical information considered essential for understanding the rationale of the procedures has been included. Methods of eye care have not been included, since there are already a number of excellent guides covering this area.

It should be realized that this guide is not intended to provide an exhaustive review of techniques in disability prevention; however, it does highlight the essential principles of disability prevention in patients with leprosy and describes various simple techniques that can be adapted to meet local needs. It is hoped that, with increasing practical field experience, it will be possible to improve our techniques in disability prevention. If this guide helps in that direction, to any extent, it will have fulfilled its purpose.

Dr S. K. Noordeen
Chief Medical Officer, Leprosy Control
World Health Organization

Introduction

This is a practical guide for peripheral health personnel to help them deal with the task of preventing disabilities and deformities in leprosy patients in their care. Most leprosy patients do *not* have disabilities or deformities when the disease first appears, and develop them later. Even when patients develop disabilities and deformities, they are mild and reversible to begin with and become severe and permanent only later on. Indeed, many conditions leading to disability and deformity can be cured if action is taken at an early stage, and the development of disabilities and deformities can be prevented.

Prevention of disabilities and deformities is easier during the early stages of their development and the actions necessary for such prevention can be taken at that stage in the field, by peripheral health personnel.

> Disabilities and deformities can be prevented
> under field conditions

Disabilities and deformities progress and worsen only gradually in most patients. Timely action can prevent such worsening. Again, this can be achieved under field conditions.

> Worsening of disabilities and deformities can be
> prevented under field conditions

It is most important to realize that the peripheral worker cannot prevent disabilities in leprosy patients simply by giving them pills or distributing pamphlets among them. Disability prevention requires active collaboration between health care personnel on the one hand and patients and their families on the other. Only then can the goal of prevention of disability in leprosy patients be realized.

> Disability prevention requires health care
> personnel and patients to work together

How to achieve this goal is described in this manual. In Chapter 1 the consequences of leprosy are outlined, while Chapter 3 describes the goals and aims of disability prevention. Further details of how to achieve these goals are described in subsequent chapters, which also describe the specific actions needed to prevent disability in patients with insensitive hands and feet (Chapters 4 and 5) and to preserve nerve function (Chapter 6).

CHAPTER 1
Consequences of leprosy

1.1 Impairments

Disease produces changes in the structure and functioning of certain parts of the body. These changes are called **impairments**. In the case of leprosy they occur in: (i) the face, giving rise to facial disfigurement and deformities; (ii) the nerves, damaging their structure and function; (iii) the eyes, causing defective vision; and (iv) the minds of patients, giving rise to personality disorders. Facial disfigurement, nerve damage, eye damage and personality disorders are impairments directly resulting from leprosy.

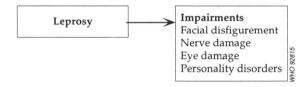

A deformity is a visible impairment or a visible consequence of an impairment inside the body.

1.2 Secondary impairments

An impairment resulting directly from a disease can itself lead to the development of further, secondary, impairments. In leprosy, the conditions grouped as "anaesthetic deformities" are secondary impairments. These are the complications that result from unprotected use of insensitive hands and feet, e.g. ulcers, stiff joints or contractures of fingers, shortening of fingers and toes, and disintegration of bones of the foot. The insensitivity in the hands and feet is due to nerve damage, which is a primary impairment, since it is a direct consequence of leprosy.

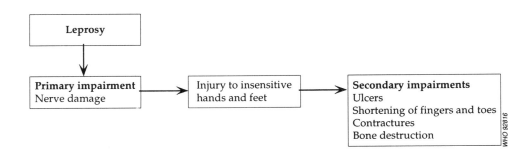

1.3 Disability

When there is an impairment (primary or secondary), the affected person finds it difficult or impossible to carry out certain activities; this is a **disability**. Leprosy patients often suffer from a variety of disabilities. For example, manual dexterity (skilful use of the hand) may be affected because of insensitivity and muscle paralysis; walking may become difficult because of ulcers or disintegration of bones of the foot; orientation in space, mobility and many other aspects of living may become difficult or impossible because the eyesight has become very poor; and behaviour may be affected by personality disorders.

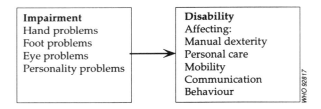

1.4 Handicaps, dehabilitation and destitution

A persistently disabled person experiences many disadvantages that limit or prevent that person from fulfilling his or her normal role in society. These disadvantages are known as **handicaps**. Leprosy patients with disabilities experience and suffer from a variety of handicaps. For example, they may lose their jobs and, therefore, their economic independence, which means that they cannot support their families. In addition, those who are severely disabled may lose their physical independence, since they need others to care for them. In some places the mere diagnosis of leprosy is sufficient to handicap the affected person, even when there is no disability.

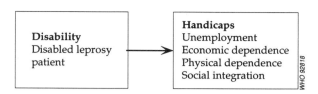

Eventually, the leprosy patient loses social status and becomes progressively isolated from society, family and friends. This is the process of dehabilitation. Dehabilitation is completed when the patient is forced to leave his or her home and settle in a rehabilitation home or in a leprosy colony with other patients. Some patients eventually find themselves completely isolated from all society and destitute (without food or shelter).

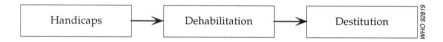

The above-mentioned consequences of leprosy are shown in a schematic form below.

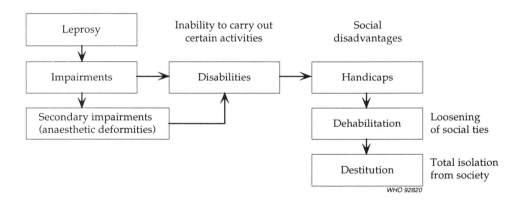

1.5 Disability prevention

For many people, leprosy is always associated with deformities. Prevention of disability involves prevention of impairments and so of deformities as well, and their worsening. By successfully implementing disability prevention, and by helping patients to overcome their disabilities, health workers can prevent them from becoming handicapped and dehabilitated.

CHAPTER 2

Nerve trunk involvement and its consequences

2.1 Stages of nerve involvement

Most disability problems in leprosy patients occur because nerve trunks are affected by the disease. The affected nerves may be in the stage of involvement, stage of damage, or stage of destruction.

Stage of involvement

At the stage of involvement the affected nerve trunk is thicker than normal (nerve thickening) and it may be painful to touch (nerve tenderness). There may also be spontaneous pain (nerve pain) of varying severity. However, there is no evidence of loss of function, e.g. anaesthesia or muscle weakness.

I Stage of involvement

- Thickening of nerve
- Tenderness
- Pain
- No loss of function

Stage of damage

When an involved nerve trunk becomes damaged, its functions are affected. The area of skin supplied by the nerve does not sweat (loss of sweating) and cannot feel (loss of sensibility or sensory loss or anaesthesia). If the affected nerve also supplies some muscles, they become weak or paralysed (motor paralysis). These signs indicate that the nerve trunk is getting damaged or paralysed.

The stage of damage is diagnosed when there is incomplete nerve paralysis or when the nerve trunk has been completely paralysed for not more than 6–9 months.

II Stage of damage

- Loss of sweating
- Loss of sensibility
- Muscle weakness
- Incomplete paralysis or recent complete paralysis
- Recovery possible

Nerve paralysis is said to be incomplete:

— when sensations are still felt in some areas of skin supplied by the affected nerve;
— when the loss of sensibility is partial, affecting only certain types of sensations;
— when some of the muscles supplied by the affected nerve are not completely paralysed.

Nerve paralysis is said to be complete:

— when the entire area of skin supplied by the affected nerve shows loss of sensibility;
— when the loss of sensibility is total, affecting all types of sensations;
— when all the muscles supplied by the nerve are completely paralysed.

It is important to recognize the stage of nerve damage because these nerves can recover with treatment. By treating patients at this stage, you can prevent permanent nerve paralysis and prevent permanent disability and deformity.

Stage of destruction

This is the end stage when the damaged nerve has been completely destroyed. At this stage, even with treatment, the nerve cannot recover function to any useful degree. This stage is diagnosed when the nerve has been completely paralysed for at least one year.

III Stage of destruction

- Complete nerve paralysis present for at least one year
- Nerve is destroyed
- No recovery possible

The above information regarding the different stages of affection of nerves in leprosy patients is summarized in the scheme shown below.

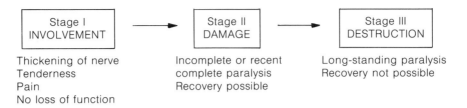

| Stage I INVOLVEMENT | Stage II DAMAGE | Stage III DESTRUCTION |

Thickening of nerve
Tenderness
Pain
No loss of function

Incomplete or recent
complete paralysis
Recovery possible

Long-standing paralysis
Recovery not possible

2.2 Types of nerves affected

Three kinds of nerves are affected in leprosy patients. They are: (i) *dermal nerves*, which are very fine nerves in the skin; (ii) *cutaneous nerves*, which are thicker nerves that run just under the skin; and (iii) *major nerve trunks*, which are large nerves. From the point of view of disability and deformity, damage to nerve trunks is far more important than damage to dermal or cutaneous nerves.

The nerve trunks commonly affected in leprosy are shown in Fig. 1. The nerves supplying the hands and feet are frequently affected and that is the reason why these parts are often the sites of impairments and deformities which cause disability.

2.3 Effects of damage to nerve trunks

Composition of nerve trunks

Nerve trunks are mixed nerves, that is they carry nerve fibres supplying the skin as well as those supplying muscles. These fibres convey messages or signals: (i) from the skin to the brain, providing the ability to feel sensations in the skin (sensibility); (ii) from the brain to the sweat glands in the skin, stimulating these glands to function and keep the skin moist and supple; and (iii) from the brain to the muscles, stimulating the muscles to function (Fig. 2).

Effects of damage to nerve trunks

When a nerve trunk is damaged at a particular site, messages do not pass across the damaged site. This means that the normal communication between the brain and an area of skin as well as a group of muscles is

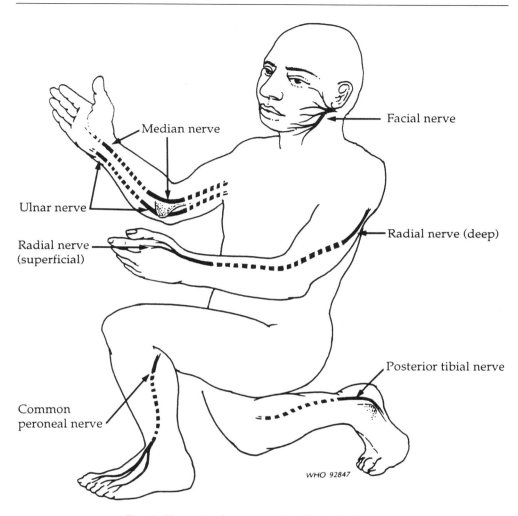

Fig. 1. Nerve trunks commonly affected in leprosy

interrupted. This results in: (i) impairment of sensibility over the area of skin supplied by the nerve trunk, because messages from the skin do not reach the brain; (ii) dryness of the skin, because messages from the brain do not reach the sweat glands; and (iii) weakness or paralysis of the muscles supplied by the nerve trunk and paralytic deformities, because messages from the brain do not reach the muscles (Fig. 3).

Impairment of sensibility

Sensibility is the ability to feel sensations in the skin. When a nerve trunk is damaged, this ability is altered, giving rise to: (i) abnormal sensations,

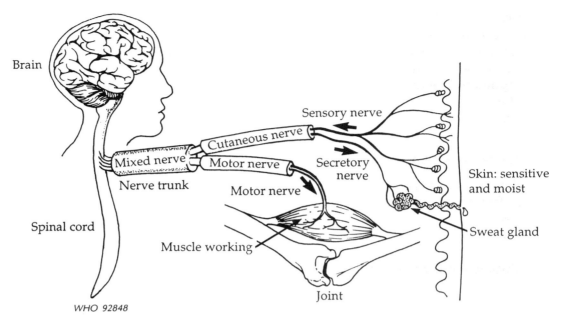

Fig. 2. A normal nerve trunk

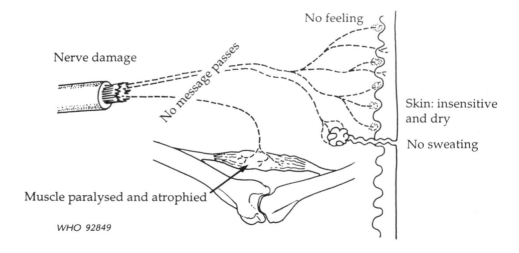

Fig. 3. A damaged nerve trunk

e.g. hypersensitive skin, burning sensations, numbness and tingling sensations; (ii) dryness of the skin supplied by the nerve; and (iii) loss of
sensibility or inability to feel in the affected skin. In the early stages of
nerve damage, only part of the area supplied by the nerve becomes dry and

loses sensibility. In addition, the loss of sensibility affects only some modalities (e.g. pain, temperature), but not others (e.g. light touch, pressure), i.e. there is incomplete loss of sensibility. Later, the ability to feel all sensations, including touch, is lost and the entire area of skin supplied by the nerve becomes completely insensitive or anaesthetic. Fig. 4 shows which areas of skin of the palms and soles are affected in the case of damage to different nerves.

Muscle weakness and paralytic deformity

When a nerve trunk is damaged, the nerve supply to the muscles may also be affected, usually some time after the supply to the skin is affected. The muscles initially become weak and later paralysed, giving rise to paralytic deformities.

Joints are normally held in balance by the forces produced by muscles around the joint (Fig. 5(a)). Paralysis of some muscles upsets this balance of forces around the joints moved by these muscles and those joints move into new positions because of the changed disposition of forces (Fig. 5(b)). These new positions or postures of the joints are seen as deformities. For example, when the ulnar nerve is paralysed, the muscles around the finger joints, especially those of the little and ring fingers, become paralysed. This upsets the balance of forces around these joints and they become bent, giving rise to the claw deformity (Fig. 6).

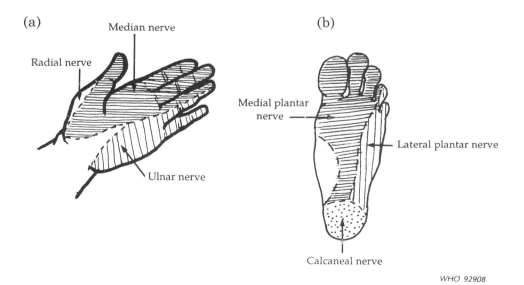

WHO 92908

Fig. 4. Site of sensory loss in the palm and sole in the case of damage to different nerves

Because each nerve trunk supplies a different set of muscles, damage to a nerve trunk gives rise to a distinctive type of paralytic deformity, from which it is possible to identify which nerve trunk has been damaged. In leprosy, certain nerve trunks become damaged more often than others and so some paralytic deformities are seen more commonly than others. The nerve trunks frequently damaged in leprosy and the resulting deformities are shown in the table below.

Nerve trunk damaged	Deformity
Ulnar nerve	Claw fingers
Median nerve	Claw thumb
Radial nerve	Drop-wrist
Common peroneal nerve	Drop-foot
Posterior tibial nerve	Claw toes
Facial nerve	Lagophthalmos

Secondary impairments following nerve trunk damage

Secondary impairments are those that occur as a consequence of primary impairments. In leprosy, the secondary impairments (anaesthetic deformities) which occur in the hands, feet and eyes are more disabling than the primary impairments, e.g. dryness, insensitivity or paralytic deformity. However, they can be prevented more easily than primary impairments, by following certain procedures (see pages 118–125).

The secondary impairments that are commonly seen in the hands and feet are listed below and are then described briefly.

Secondary impairments

1. Cracks and wounds
2. Ulcers
3. Septic hand or foot
4. Joint stiffness or contractures
5. Shortening of fingers or toes
6. Mutilation of the hand or foot
7. Disorganization of the foot or wrist

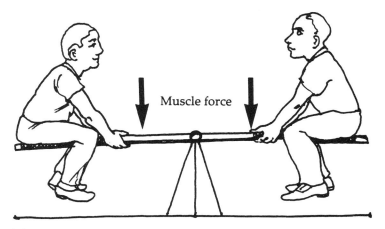

(a) Normal.
Forces balanced on both sides of the joint.

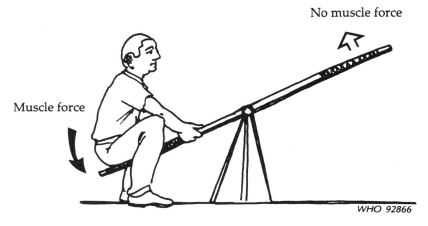

(b) Some muscles paralysed.
Balance of forces around the joint changed.
Joint moves into a new position.

Fig. 5. Effect of paralysis of muscles

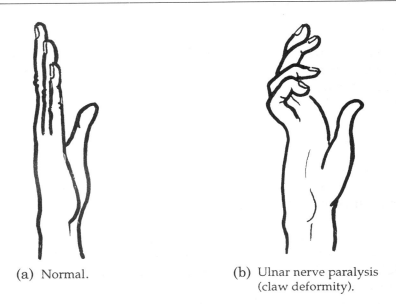

| (a) Normal. | (b) Ulnar nerve paralysis (claw deformity). |

Fig. 6. Deformity of the hand due to paralysis of the ulnar nerve

Cracks and wounds

Long-standing dryness of the skin makes it less supple and more brittle than normal skin which has been kept moist by sweating. The brittle, dry skin breaks where it is repeatedly bent and straightened (e.g. in front of a finger joint), and the patient develops a *skin crack*. Insensitive skin does not register pain when it is injured, therefore the injury is neglected. Burns, cuts and other wounds occurring in insensitive hands and feet are often neglected for the same reason.

Ulcers

As the patient does not feel pain, the wounds and cracks are neglected and they do not heal. Instead, they become ulcers. Ulcers may also arise because of repeated excessive pressure over certain parts of the anaesthetic foot or hand. In the foot these excessive pressures occur during walking, when there is some abnormality such as deformity or muscle paralysis. This kind of internal injury also causes breakdown of tissue under the skin and formation of a blister, which breaks open to form an ulcer. This kind of ulcer is seen most often in the sole of the foot and is known as a plantar ulcer.

Septic hand or foot

Severe and gross infection may complicate a skin crack, wound or ulcer, causing widespread tissue damage and acute inflammation in the affected part. When this occurs, the part is said to be septic. This can happen in the hand or the foot.

Joint stiffness

Tissues damaged by injury or infection heal with the formation of scars. Scars located close to joints and those that involve tendons prevent joint movement and the joint becomes stiff. A joint also becomes stiff if it is not regularly moved through its full range of motion. For example, if a joint is kept bent for some time, the loose tissue on the bent side does not get stretched and eventually the tissue becomes shortened. The joint cannot be straightened at that stage because the shortened tissue does not permit the joint to be opened up. This type of joint stiffness is called a contracture or fixed deformity. Fingers and even the whole foot can develop contractures in this manner.

Shortening of digits

As mentioned above, tissues may be damaged or destroyed by infection or injury. Dead tissue may be eliminated by the body by normal (physiological) mechanisms or be removed by surgery. In leprosy, bones and parts of the fingers or toes may be lost in either of these ways, resulting in shortening of the digits.

Mutilation of the hand or foot

When many digits are severely shortened, the hand or foot may become a stump and appear mutilated.

Disorganization of the foot or wrist

Sometimes one or more bones of the foot get broken up as a result of an injury or weakening of the bone from infection or disuse. Since this is not associated with pain, the patient continues to walk and otherwise use the foot as if it were normal. The bone damage spreads and eventually the bones of the foot disintegrate, that is, the foot becomes disorganized. The wrist may also become disorganized in this manner.

CHAPTER 3
Disability prevention

3.1 Goals and aims of disability prevention

The goals of a disability prevention programme are: (i) to prevent the occurrence of any disability or deformity not already present at the time when the disease is diagnosed; and (ii) to prevent the worsening of existing disabilities and deformities.

> No new disabilities or deformities
> No worsening of existing disabilities or deformities

Achieving these goals will require a series of appropriate actions with clear and well-defined aims. These aims are:

— to protect and preserve insensitive (and possibly deformed) hands;
— to protect and preserve insensitive (and possibly deformed) feet;
— to protect eyes from damage and preserve eyesight;
— to preserve nerve function.

The health worker as well as the patient will have to take a number of actions in order to achieve the above four aims. These actions are discussed below.

3.2 Actions by health care workers

The health care worker has six main tasks to perform in order to achieve the goal of disability prevention. These tasks have to be carried out systematically, taking into consideration the relevant condition and the needs of individual patients. The six tasks are listed below and are discussed in greater detail in the subsequent sections of this chapter.

Actions by health care workers

1. Assess and record the risk status of each patient.
2. Assess and record the disability status.
3. Treat treatable conditions.
4. Instruct and train patients in disability prevention.
5. Monitor and support patients.
6. Refer patients to appropriate centres for further care.

Assess and record the risk status of the patient

Not all leprosy patients will develop disabilities and deformities. Some are more likely to develop them than are others. Of these, some will be in great danger of developing further problems and will require urgent specific action. Therefore the risk status of all patients at the start of the disability prevention programme and all new patients thereafter should be assessed by clinical examination and questioning, as outlined below.

1. Ask for history of any previous problems:

    — eye problems;
    — hand problems;
    — foot problems;
    — nerve problems;
    — reactions.

2. Examine for presence of any problems:

    — loss of sensibility in hands or feet;
    — thickening of nerve trunks (number of nerve trunks involved, level of tenderness);
    — deformities of hands or feet;
    — changes in eyes;
    — weakness of eyelid muscles.

3. Consider the overall picture:

    — type of disease;
    — extent of disease;
    — other factors, e.g. occupation, treatment.

"In danger" group. Patients who have already developed some impairments and disabilities are in great danger of developing new disabilities as well as worsening of existing ones and need urgent specific action. If any of the following characteristics are present, the patient should be assigned to the "in danger" group.

Characteristic	Comment
Past or present eye problem Weakness of eyelid muscles	Danger of eye damage and loss of sight
Anaesthesia of hand (palmar surface) Past or present ulceration or crack in hand Deformities in hand	Danger of damage to hand
Anaesthesia of sole Drop-foot or other deformities in foot Past or present ulcer or crack in sole	Danger of damage to foot
Acute or subacute neuritis of a nerve trunk Incomplete or recent neural deficit	Danger of permanent damage to nerve

---

In danger

Patients who already have some impairment
involving the eyes, hands, feet or nerve trunks

"At-risk" group. Patients who have not yet developed impairments or disabilities but who show any of the following characteristics should be assigned to the "at-risk" group. Such patients are more likely to develop problems and disabilities than those in the "low-risk" group and need to be monitored. Remember that, in many cases, the risk of nerve damage is greater during the first 6–12 months after starting anti-leprosy treatment.

Characteristic	Comment
Multibacillary leprosy Multiple skin patches Three or more thickened nerve trunks Moderate or severe tenderness of a nerve trunk Past or present reactions Pregnancy (with or without thickened nerve trunks)	Increased risk of damage to eyes, hands, feet and nerves and their consequences compared with patients in the "low-risk" group

---

At risk

Patients with extensive disease,
many nerve trunks thickened,
or a history of reactions,
and patients who are pregnant

"Low-risk" group. Patients with the following characteristics and patients who are not included in either of the two previous categories should be assigned to the "low-risk" group. The likelihood of disability is low in these patients and they need only occasional checking.

Characteristic	Comment
Paucibacillary leprosy with few skin patches	Likelihood of disability is low in these patients

The risk status for disability must be periodically reassessed and revised as necessary. The clinical situation may change (e.g. increase in or onset of anaesthesia or muscle weakness; diminution in visual acuity; or increase in or onset of nerve tenderness with neuritis or reactions) and then the risk status may also change. Therefore, it is important to update the risk status periodically. For this, teach the patient to report: (a) any eye problems; (b) any change in sensibility in the hands or feet; (c) any change in muscle strength in the hands or feet; and (d) any change in symptoms relating to the nerve trunks.

At every clinical assessment, reassess the risk for disability, compare the findings with the results of the previous assessment and decide whether or not the risk status needs to be revised.

Record the current risk status of the patient, and the type of risk prominently in the case chart and the patient register. Use special stickers, rubber stamps or coloured tabs or symbols to indicate whether further action is required.

Assess and record the disability status

The disability status of the patient must also be assessed periodically. In these assessments, check the following:

● State of eyes:

— eyelids;
— cornea;
— conjunctiva;
— pupils;
— vision;
— muscles of the eyelids.

- State of nerve trunks:
  - ulnar nerves at elbow and wrist;
  - median nerves at elbow and wrist;
  - common peroneal nerves behind knee;
  - posterior tibial nerves behind ankle.

- State of hands and feet:
  - sensibility;
  - ulcers, skin cracks, scars and callosities;
  - deformity;
  - muscle strength.

Record the results in a special disability chart and compare them with the previous findings. Patients in the "in danger" group will need immediate attention.

Treat treatable conditions

Many potentially dangerous conditions (e.g. acute neuritis, ulcers, skin cracks, recent muscle paralysis and eye problems) can be satisfactorily treated in the field and prevented from worsening. Details of simple methods of treatment are given in Chapters 4–6. If the patient has a condition that needs immediate attention and care that is not available at your level, he or she must be sent to the nearest referral facility.

Instruct and train patients

Patients in the "at-risk" group or the "in danger" group need to be instructed in disability prevention. Details of practices to prevent disabilities are given in Chapter 7. The instructions may be given collectively to groups of patients with similar problems as well as to individual patients according to their special needs. At least one person from the patient's family will also need to be instructed and trained about the problem and methods of preventing disability.

Make the instructions clear, simple and easy to understand. Avoid using jargon. The instructions should include:

- a description of the problem the patient faces;
- the consequences of the problem;
- the reasons for preventive practices;
- a description and demonstration of the practices.

For instructions to be successful you must:

— organize the instruction sessions in a systematic manner;
— avoid irrelevant details;
— use familiar examples and illustrative aids;
— use intelligible language;
— let patients comment and ask questions;
— go step by step, ensuring that patients understand what you have told them before you proceed further.

Disability prevention depends, to a very large extent, on the patient. For example, a patient with insensitive hands or feet has to become aware of anaesthesia of the extremities as a disability and the consequences of unprotected use of insensitive hands and feet. The patient has to learn how to avoid those consequences. The patient has to practise what has been learnt and this requires training.

The patient needs to be trained in the following:

— to recognize at an early stage: injury and inflammation, changes in sensibility, onset of muscle weakness, and worsening of visual acuity;
— to deal with simple problems and to report complex or persistent ones;
— to take care of insensitive and dry eyes;
— to protect insensitive hands and feet from injuries;
— to take care of dry skin of hands and feet;
— to take care of wounds, ulcers and skin cracks in hands and feet;
— to practise oil massage and exercises at home;
— to take care of footwear, aids and appliances.

In all these areas, simple instruction alone is not enough. Each procedure must be demonstrated several times. The patient should then practise the procedures under supervision until he or she can perform them correctly. Ideally, a family member or friend of the patient and some volunteers from the community should also be trained in these procedures.

Monitor and support patients

Monitoring the patient is an essential feature of the disability prevention programme. Monitoring has two aspects: (i) monitoring the clinical picture by periodic reassessment (see page 19); and (ii) monitoring the practices of the patient. The objectives of the latter are:

— to help the patient continue to practise self-care activities to prevent disabilities;

— to see that the patient practises them correctly;
— to help the patient overcome any social, cultural or economic obstacles that may prevent him or her from practising the activities.

The patient should also be provided with footwear and other aids and appliances as required and encouraged to practise self-care activities. Above all, you should help the patient to lead as normal a life as possible, in spite of having some disabilities, and to live without developing further disabilities.

3.3 Actions by patients

Ultimately, it is the patient who becomes disabled and deformed, and if disabilities and deformities are to be avoided, the patient has to participate actively as an equal partner in the programme. Patients must learn:

— to recognize the signs of onset or worsening of impairments and take appropriate action;
— to practise hand care;
— to practise foot care;
— to practise care of the eyes.

Further details of these actions are given at appropriate places in Chapters 4–7.

3.4 Summary

The activities involved in disability prevention are summarized in the table opposite.

Activity	Aim
Assess patient	To determine risk status for disability
Record risk status	To identify patients requiring treatment
Record disability status	To provide clinical picture for comparison
Treat problems	To prevent worsening
Instruct patient	To improve patient understanding
Train patient	To ensure that patient learns practices to prevent disabilities
Monitor patient	To ensure that patient practises disability prevention and that he or she does so correctly
Support patient	To help patient lead a normal life

CHAPTER 4
Preventing damage to insensitive hands

In this chapter the specific actions needed to prevent secondary impairments occurring in insensitive hands and to prevent existing injuries from worsening are described.

4.1 Examine to ascertain the risk status

Do a rapid and systematic screening examination of the hands of all patients at the beginning of the disability prevention programme, and of all new patients thereafter. The aim of this examination is to assess the sensibility of the hands and the condition of the skin, and to detect any deformities or stiffness of the joints.

Sensibility testing

Ask the patient whether he or she can feel pain, heat, touch and pressure, everywhere in the hand. Test for perception of pain (using a pin), touch (using a feather or a nylon filament), pressure (using a blunt point, e.g. a ball-point pen) and, if feasible, for perception of heat. Test the five sites shown in Fig. 7.

Impaired sensibility is identified if perception of any of these sensations is diminished or lost in any of the sites tested.

Skin condition

Examine the hands for blisters, scars, ulcers, wounds, cracks or callosities (localized hardening or thickening of the skin).

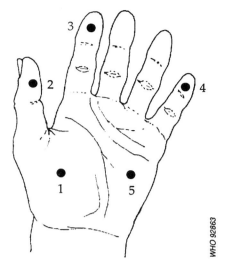

1. Thenar eminence, about 1.0–1.5 cm from the crease at the base of the thumb, along a line extending from the midline of the thumb.
2. Pulp of the thumb.
3. Pulp of the index finger.
4. Pulp of the little finger.
5. Palm, about 3-4 cm from the crease at the base of the little finger, along a line extending from the midline of the finger.

Fig. 7. Sites for testing sensibility

Stiffness of joints

Try to straighten out all the joints of the patient's hands and fingers, without using force. If force is needed, or any joint of the patient's fingers cannot be straightened out, that joint has stiffness.

Deformity

See whether the patient can open out and spread all the fingers and thumb of each hand and keep them straight without any help from the other hand. If that is not possible, or there is noticeable shortening of a digit, there is a deformity.

4.2 Assignment of risk status

If any of the following conditions are present, the hand should be categorized as being "in danger": (i) blisters, ulcers, scars, cracks or wounds; (ii) deformity; (iii) swelling; and (iv) muscle wasting.

When there is only loss of sensibility, without any other change, there is a risk of the hand getting injured (and injuries being neglected) during routine activities such as cooking and washing of clothes and utensils, as well as at work, during recreational activities or by accident. Therefore, the hand should be categorized as being "at risk".

If none of the above conditions is present, the hand should be categorized as having "no risk at present". The criteria for determining the risk status and nature of risk are summarized in the table below.

Condition	Risk status and nature of risk
Normal sensibility	No risk at present
Only impaired sensibility (no other abnormality)	At risk of injuries, burns, etc.
Blisters, ulcers, scars, cracks, wounds, deformity, swelling or muscle wasting	In danger of progressive damage and disability

4.3 Record the risk status of the hand

If the hand is "in danger" or "at risk", this should be recorded prominently in the case chart and the patient register in order to indicate that further action is required. You may use a special rubber stamp, symbols or colour-coding to indicate the risk status of the hand.

4.4 Assess and record the current impairment status

The degree of impairment should also be recorded. This record is important as it shows the initial state of the hand and will be needed for future comparison. What you should record and how are shown in the following table.

Condition	Indicate by
Loss or impairment of sensibility	Slanting lines
Scars or callosities	Cross-hatching
Cracks	Lens-like figure
Blisters	"B" enclosed in a circle
Ulcers	Two concentric circles. Indicate size, state (clean or dirty, etc.) and duration
Deformity	"C" for clawing. Indicate degree of clawing, if feasible Indicate level of shortening by " = " sign across the digit
Stiffness	Indicate in writing
Swelling	Indicate in writing
Muscle wasting	Indicate in writing

A sample current impairment status record for the hand is shown below (Fig. 8).

To assess the extent of impairment of sensibility, you should examine and test a number of sites (not just the five sites shown in Fig. 7) in the palm and palmar surface of the fingers and thumb.

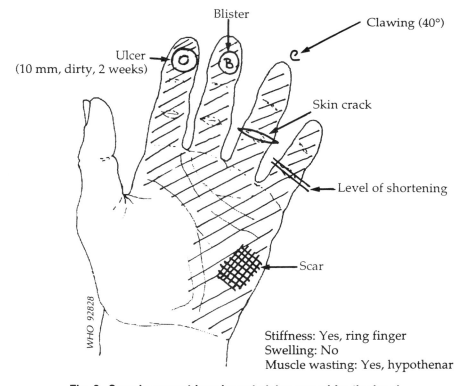

Blister

Clawing (40°)

Ulcer
(10 mm, dirty, 2 weeks)

Skin crack

Level of shortening

Scar

WHO 92828

Stiffness: Yes, ring finger
Swelling: No
Muscle wasting: Yes, hypothenar

Fig. 8. Sample current impairment status record for the hand

4.5 Treat treatable conditions

Conditions noted at the time of the initial assessment, or at any other time later, need to be treated to prevent them worsening. All these conditions can be treated at your level, provided they are identified early.

Treat at your level

skin cracks, blisters, callosities, wounds, swelling, ulcers, and deformities, to prevent worsening of disabilities

---

If the above conditions are not treated, they will become worse and the hand will become stiff, deformed and disabled.

Priorities

Hands with acute inflammation should be treated immediately. The inflammation is usually caused by infection. If treatment is delayed, the infection and inflammation will spread, causing widespread tissue destruction, and the hand will become stiff, deformed and disabled.

Prompt treatment is also required if a deformity develops, to prevent the hands becoming stiff.

However, hands that are already very stiff or that have grossly shortened fingers will not improve very much, even with intensive treatment. Therefore, they have a lower priority for treatment, unless there is acute inflammation.

Raw areas in the hand

Ulcers, wounds and skin cracks in the hand are collectively called "raw areas". Raw areas may be:

— small or large;
— recent or long-standing (chronic);
— superficial or deep;
— simple or complicated;
— relatively clean or septic and acutely inflamed.

A raw area is *superficial* if it involves only the skin and the tissue immediately under the skin (Fig. 9(a)). *Deep* raw areas extend below the

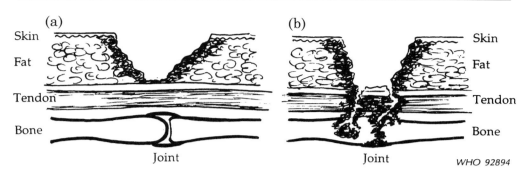

Fig. 9. Raw areas

skin; in many cases, they are also *complicated*, because structures such as tendons, bones and joints are affected (Fig. 9(b)). These structures are not affected in a simple raw area. Fig. 10 shows an example of a complicated ulcer in the hand. The ulcer is also *dirty*, because there is some discharge of pus and the finger is swollen. The infection has spread from the finger to the palm. Early treatment of the wound would have prevented this complication.

A *relatively clean* raw area has some discharge of bloodstained fluid, but no discharge of pus. When there is much discharge of foul-smelling pus and the affected part, or even the whole hand, is swollen, the raw area is *septic*. Often there is also some pain. The lymph glands in the armpit may be tender and swollen and fever may also be present.

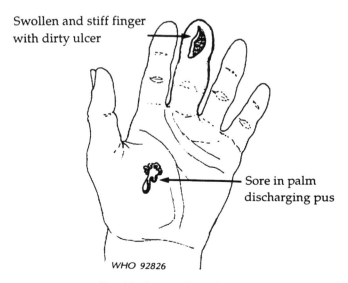

Fig. 10. A complicated ulcer

Septic raw areas need immediate treatment, otherwise they can lead to severe disabilities and deformities. It is best to refer patients with septic raw areas for special treatment.

The principles of management of a raw area in the hand are the same, whether the raw area is an ulcer, wound or skin crack. They are:

— to clean the raw area — to remove dirt and infection;
— to cover it — to keep it clean;
— to rest the affected part — to allow healing.

Cleaning

Wash the whole hand well with soapy water. Scrub the skin of the hand with a piece of cloth or soft brush to remove all dirt, but do not rub the raw area itself. Carefully remove all foreign bodies such as sand, gravel, splinters of wood or metal and any other dirt with clean forceps.

Dry the hand well using a clean cloth or towel. Do not rub the raw area, but mop it dry. Do *not* use cotton wool to dry the raw area.

Covering

If the raw area is simple, relatively clean and superficial, cover it and the surrounding skin with strips of ordinary zinc oxide sticking plaster. The strips should be 5–8 mm wide. Apply the plaster strips directly over the raw area, ensuring that each strip overlaps the previous one by 2–3 mm (Fig. 11).

If sticking plaster is not available, use two layers of clean (sterile, if possible) gauze or cloth to cover the raw area. There is usually no need to apply local medications. However, if there is some discharge from the raw area, the gauze or cloth may stick to the raw area. This can be prevented by applying an antiseptic ointment or using gauze or cloth soaked in sterile petroleum jelly, liquid paraffin or oil. Place a few layers of soft clean cloth or clean cotton wool on top of this dressing and cover with a bandage to keep the dressing in place.

When you are bandaging raw areas in the finger, do *not* tie the bandage at the base of the finger (Fig. 12(a)). Instead, carry the bandage over to the palm and tie it with a knot on the back of the hand (Fig. 12(b)). Alternatively you can use sticking plaster to secure the bandage.

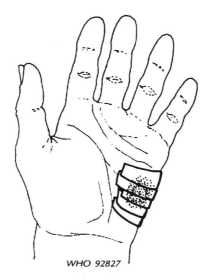

WHO 92827

Fig. 11. Dressing a raw area in the hand using sticking plaster

Note the following points:

1. Leave the fingertip and a portion of the nail exposed, unless the raw area is on the fingertip. If the bandage is too tight, or if there is a lot of swelling, the blood supply to the finger will be affected and it will turn white (pale) or blue. If the fingertip is covered, it will not be possible to see this colour change. Therefore, leave the fingertip exposed.
2. Tell the patient to remove the bandage immediately if the fingertip becomes blue or pale.
3. Do not use rubber bands to secure the bandage. They may cut off the blood supply to the finger.
4. For the same reason, do not tie the bandage at the base of the finger. Take the bandage around the palm a few times (or, in the case of the thumb, around the wrist) and tie the knot over the back of the hand. Alternatively, use a piece of sticking plaster to secure the finger bandage.

If the raw area is deep:

(i) Cover it with gauze, cloth or sticking plaster as described above;
(ii) On top of it, pack the wound with loosely rolled-up gauze, cloth or cotton wool to fit snugly into the area, such that the top of the pack is level with the skin surface;

(a) Wrong

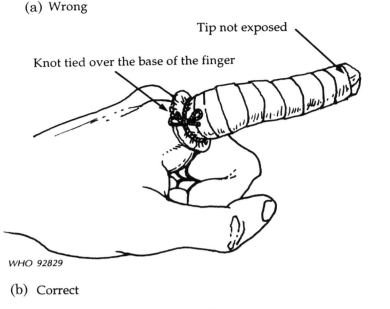

Tip not exposed

Knot tied over the base of the finger

WHO 92829

(b) Correct

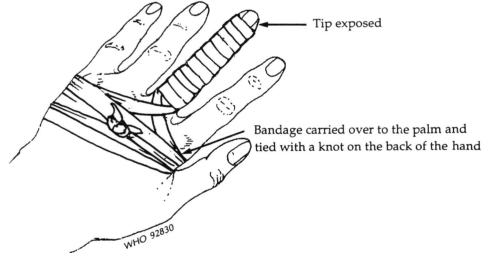

Tip exposed

Bandage carried over to the palm and tied with a knot on the back of the hand

WHO 92830

Fig. 12. Applying finger bandages

(iii) Put a second layer of gauze or sticking plaster on top to keep the pack in place (see Fig. 13). If gauze or pieces of cloth are used, put a bandage on top of the dressing.

Care of bandage: The aim of covering the raw area is to prevent it becoming contaminated. This will not be achieved if the bandage gets wet

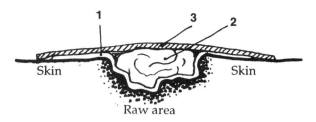

1. Layer of gauze, cloth or sticking plaster.
2. Rolled-up gauze, cloth or cotton wool to fill the depression.
3. Top layer of gauze or sticking plaster.

WHO 92895

Fig. 13. Dressing deeper raw areas

or very dirty, or becomes displaced. So, instruct the patient:

— to avoid wetting the bandage (e.g. when bathing, wrap the hand in a plastic bag and keep it out of the water);
— to avoid dirtying the bandage, to the extent possible;
— if the bandage gets displaced, to put it on properly without delay; and
— if it gets wet, to remove the dressing, clean the affected part, dry it and apply a fresh dressing and bandage.

Sticking plaster is waterproof and even if it gets wet, water is unlikely to reach the wound, so very strict precautions against wetting are not necessary. However, when the raw area gets wet, it should be dried promptly.

Teach the patient and a family member how to dress the wound and apply the sticking plaster or bandages. Provide the patient with some spare dressings, if possible. In any case, *every patient with insensitive hands should always keep some sticking plaster, a few pieces of clean gauze or cloth and some bandaging material.*

Resting

A raw area in the hand will heal only if it is allowed to heal. If it is frequently pressed upon, moved, rubbed or subjected to other physical damage, healing will be delayed. So the affected part must be rested, preferably by splinting.

For raw areas in the fingers, use a finger splint. It can be made from any smooth, stiff material, e.g. cardboard, wood, metal or plastic. Even a few matchsticks tied or glued together can be used as a finger splint. However, it is better to use splints made from thick-walled (3 mm) rubber or plastic tubing (see Fig. 14). These splints are safe and washable. *Prepare and keep a few such splints in stock.*

The points to note are:

1. The edges of the splint should be smooth and not sharp.
2. The splint should be padded along the edges and at the base, where it touches the palm (Fig. 15).
3. The splint should be held in place with a bandage or sticking plaster. If a bandage is used, it should be secure, but not too tight. Otherwise the splint will damage the tissues of the finger.
4. The fingertip and part of the nail should be left exposed, so that the finger can be inspected for colour changes (see page 31).
5. The splint should extend into the palm for a short distance (about 2 cm). Otherwise it will dig into the palm at the base of the finger.

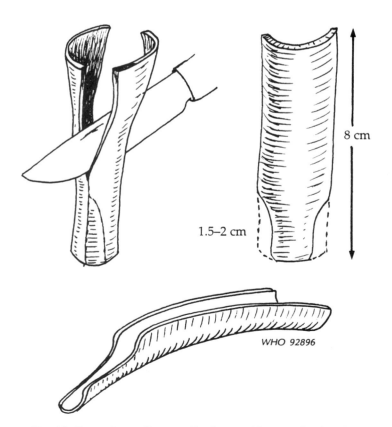

8 cm

1.5–2 cm

WHO 92896

Fig. 14. Preparing a finger splint from rubber or plastic tubing

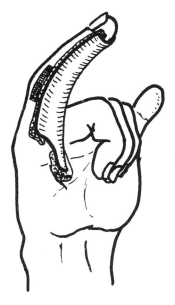

Fig. 15. Applying a finger splint

A splint to prevent too much bending of the finger during healing is necessary while treating cracks in the finger. Otherwise the crack will heal with the finger in the bent position, giving a short scar across the finger joint which will prevent later straightening of the finger (Fig. 16(a)). Furthermore, if the finger is now straightened, the short scar will break and the crack will reappear (Fig. 16(b)).

For relatively clean raw areas in the palm, splinting is not essential. Nevertheless, the raw area should be protected with dressings and bandages and the hand should not be used for rough, heavy work until it has healed properly.

(a) (b)

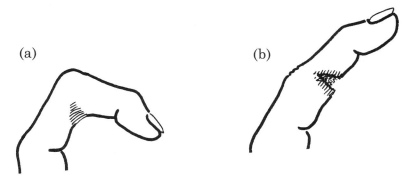

Fig. 16. A short scar breaks on straightening the finger

How often to dress the raw area

Relatively clean raw areas need not be dressed daily unless the dressing becomes wet, dirty or displaced. If sticking plaster has been used, leave it in place until it becomes loose or discharge from the raw area soaks through. Then remove the sticking plaster, clean the raw area, dry it and apply fresh strips of plaster. If gauze or cloth bandage and dressing have been used, change the dressing:

— if it gets wet or discharge from the raw area has soaked through;
— if the bandage has become loose and is displaced; or
— at least every 3–4 days.

Healing

Relatively clean raw areas should heal within 10–20 days or less, provided they are kept clean, covered and rested. Signs of healing are:

— the raw area becomes smaller and less deep;
— there is less discharge;
— any swelling subsides.

If there are no signs of healing by that time, this indicates that either there is some complication that has been missed, or the part is not being rested or covered properly. Ask the patient about both aspects and take appropriate action, such as re-examining the patient, repeating instructions and checking that the patient has understood them, and demonstrating the correct technique for dressing the raw area and ensuring that the patient does it correctly. If complications such as bone or tendon involvement are suspected, refer the patient for further examination and treatment.

Thinning edges of cracks

When the edges of the raw area are very thickened, healing is delayed. Earlier healing will occur if the edges are thinned out by cutting away the thickened superficial layers of skin. Use a sterile scalpel blade or sharp pointed stout scissors for doing this. Hold the middle of the curved blade or tips of the scissors parallel to the skin surface and cut the skin as shown in Fig. 17. If this is done properly, there should be no bleeding. Teach the patient and a family member how to do this.

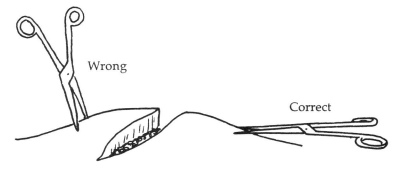

Fig. 17. Thinning edges of cracks

Septic raw areas

Septic raw areas in the hand require immediate treatment. Patients with septic raw areas must be referred for the pus to be removed, the wound cleaned, and appropriate drug treatment to control the infection. Treatment can then be continued at clinic or home level, along the same lines as for relatively clean raw areas (see page 30), except that more frequent dressing will be needed. The hand should be rested in a sling. If bulky dressings are used, it will not be necessary to splint the hand. In the case of ulcers in the palm, however, it may be more comfortable for the patient if a forearm splint, which supports the wrist while leaving the fingers and thumb free to move, is worn (Fig. 18).

A piece of light wooden board or metal strip, about 5–7.5 cm wide and about 30 cm long, can be used as a forearm splint. The splint should be wrapped in soft cloth or cotton wool and bandage before it is used.

In addition, the forearm and hand should be kept raised above heart level — in a sling during waking hours and on pillows or a rolled-up sheet at night.

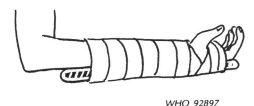

WHO 92897

Fig. 18. A forearm splint

Callosities

Sites of callosities

Callosities are localized areas of skin that have become thickened and hardened in response to repeated heavy pressure and friction. For example, manual workers often develop callosities on their hands from such pressure and friction from their work tools.

Callous areas are commonly found over the palmar surface of the fingers (usually over the middle joint), in the palm, around the base of the fingers, and in the centre of the palm (Fig. 19).

Leprosy patients with badly damaged feet often use their hands to push against the ground, for raising themselves from the sitting position (Fig. 20(a)), or for moving around in the sitting position. In such cases, callosities develop in the heel of the palm, near the wrist (Fig. 20(b)).

In insensitive hands, the skin does not sweat. The dry skin is less elastic and more brittle than normal skin. These abnormalities are increased in callous skin. This kind of skin, if it lies opposite a joint, splits open due to the repeated movement of bending and straightening the joint. This is how cracks in the fingers (and sometimes in the palm) develop.

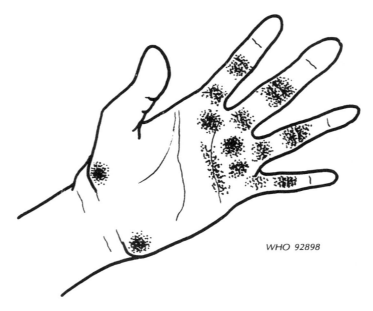

WHO 92898

Fig. 19. Common sites for callosities in the hand

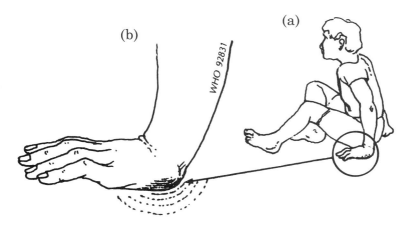

Fig. 20. Development of callosities in the "heel" of the palm

Corns are localized areas of callosity. The callosities in the heel of the palm are like corns. They can also develop into ulcers, because of injury (due to cutting too deeply into them), infection (through fine cracks or due to cutting them with an unclean knife), or pressure and friction. These ulcers do not heal easily.

It is better to *prevent* cracks and ulcers related to callosities by treating hard skin and by preventing the development of callous areas, than to treat them.

Preventing callosities

The only way to prevent the development of callous areas in insensitive hands is to avoid subjecting them to repeated localized heavy pressure and friction. For example, soft material placed between a tool handle and the hand will reduce localized pressure and friction. The material can be attached to the handle of the tool or wrapped around the hand itself.

Treating hard thick skin

Skin can be kept soft and supple by proper *skin care*. This consists of:

1. *Soaking the hand* in soapy or salty water for 15–20 minutes.
2. *Rubbing* hard skin away with a rough cloth or stone, or rubbing one palm against the other in order to remove the superficial layers of skin.
3. *Massaging* the skin with oil, without drying the skin.

4. *Applying softening ointments.* If the skin is very thick, softening ointments (e.g. salicylic acid, 5% ointment), if available, may be used. The ointment should be applied over the hard area and rubbed in well, two or three times a day. This will soften the superficial layers and they can then be removed by rubbing.

5. *Cutting away* the superficial layers of skin, using a scalpel blade or sharp pointed stout scissors. This must be done very carefully, without cutting too deep and without causing any bleeding. The instrument used must be sterile. If these conditions are not observed, a wound will be created, it will become infected and the hand will become worse than before. So, be very careful if you are cutting a corn or callosity. (See page 36 and Fig. 17 for further details.)

Swelling of the hand

A swollen hand must be treated promptly, otherwise it will become stiff and probably useless. Swelling of the hand must never be ignored.

There are three causes of swelling of the hand:

1. Infection and inflammation.
2. Injury to a bone or joint.
3. Inflammation only, without infection or injury.

If there is a raw area in the hand or a recently healed wound, and if there is increasing swelling, pain or fever, or the lymph glands in the armpit are swollen and tender, the swelling is most likely to be due to infection and inflammation. These signs indicate that an abscess is forming somewhere in the hand and the hand is becoming septic. If there is no raw area or recently healed wound, and no fever or swollen and tender glands in the armpit, the cause of swelling is most probably a closed injury, that is, an injury to a bone or joint without a break in the skin. Ask the patient for a history of the injury. When you suspect injury, examine the hand carefully, pressing each bone and joint with your fingertips. The injured part will be tender at the site of the injury.

Sometimes there may be swelling of the hand due to inflammation without injury or infection. This is not common. This kind of inflammation of the hand occurs as part of lepra reaction, an acute episode of disease in which symptoms are exacerbated. There are two main types of reaction:

— reversal reaction;
— erythema nodosum leprosum (ENL) (see page 108).

Treatment and management

Treatment of a swollen hand has two aspects: (i) finding the cause of swelling (infection, injury, reaction); and (ii) treating the swollen hand.

Finding the cause of swelling. When you suspect that the hand is septic, refer the patient immediately for treatment to let the pus out (drain the abscess) and control the infection. In the meantime, rest the hand in a sling. If you are not sure whether the hand is septic, rest it in a sling and examine it again after 24 hours. If the swelling has increased, the hand is very likely to be septic and will require immediate treatment. If the swelling has noticeably decreased by then, it is probably due to either a minor injury or a very minor infection. In that case, the hand should continue to be rested in a sling for another 48 or 72 hours. It should heal without further treatment. However, the hand should be examined every day. If the swelling gets worse at any time during this period, refer the patient immediately for treatment of septic hand.

If you suspect that the swelling is due to injury, refer the patient immediately for further examination and treatment. In the meantime, rest the hand in a splint and a sling. If you are not sure whether the hand is injured, rest it in a splint and a sling and examine it every day, for 3–4 days. If there is a noticeable decrease in swelling and tenderness, it is probably a case of minor injury; the hand should continue to be rested. If there is no or some improvement in swelling, but no significant improvement in tenderness, the hand is probably injured and you should refer the patient for further examination and treatment.

When you suspect that the swelling is due to reaction, refer the patient to persons trained to treat this condition.

Treating the swollen hand. Once the cause of swelling has been found, the swollen hand must be treated. The aims of treating the hand are:

1. To bring down the swelling as quickly as possible.
2. To prevent the hand becoming stiff.

The swelling may be reduced by:

1. Treating the cause of swelling (e.g. injury, infection, inflammation).
2. Resting the hand in a splint.
3. Keeping the hand above heart level.

The hand should be kept in the position of function, as if it is holding a thick pen (Fig. 21(a)). Any object of a suitable size may be used to hold the

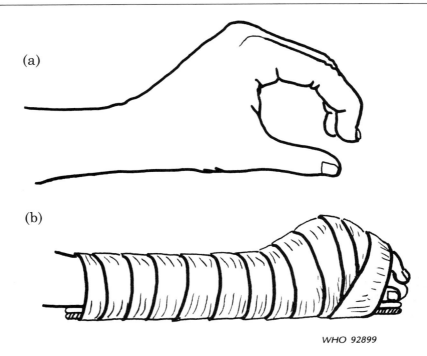

(a)

(b)

WHO 92899

Fig. 21. Splinting the hand in the position of function

hand in the position of function, e.g. a half coconut shell or balls of paper wrapped in cloth. The splint should then be bandaged to the forearm and hand as shown (Fig. 21(b)).

Elevating the hand is as important as resting it in a splint for bringing down the swelling as quickly as possible. The patient can hold the hand at chin level, but that can be tiring. It is more comfortable to keep the hand raised above heart level using an ordinary triangular sling, as shown in Fig. 22.

The hand should be kept raised above heart level all the time. Pillows or rolled-up sheets may be used to keep the hand raised at night.

Prevention of stiffness is the goal of treating a swollen hand. Right from the beginning, the shoulder and elbow joints should be kept moving. Each movement of the shoulder and elbow should be carried out at least 15–20 times, once or twice a day. Patients should be taught all the relevant movements and shown how to practise them.

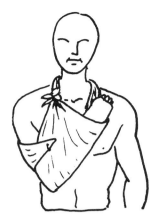

Fig. 22. Elevating the hand

The wrist and fingers should also be moved, both actively and passively. Graded exercises, starting with slight active movement and progressively increasing in range of movement, are necessary. Patients with badly swollen or septic hands will need daily supervision and monitoring of progress. You will need some training to do this.

A scheme outlining the causes and principles of management of a swollen hand is shown in Fig. 23.

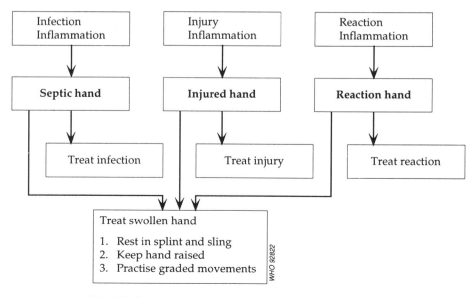

Fig. 23. Causes and management of the swollen hand

Deformity

In addition to the secondary impairments described above, leprosy patients may also have deformities of the hand, because of paralysis of muscles in the hand. Such deformities include partial claw hand deformity, in which only the fingers are affected (Fig. 24), complete claw hand deformity, in which the fingers and thumb are affected (Fig. 25), and drop-wrist, in which the fingers, thumb and wrist are affected (Fig. 26).

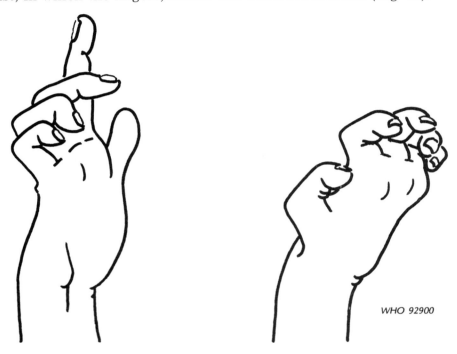

WHO 92900

Fig. 24. Partial claw hand   **Fig. 25. Complete claw hand**

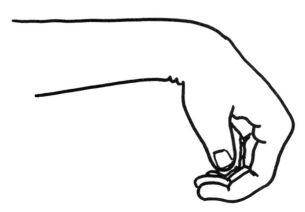

Fig. 26. Drop-wrist

These deformities can be satisfactorily corrected by surgery. However, if the hand with deformity is not properly cared for, the joints of the fingers and thumb will become stiff. Once stiffness is present, it is very difficult to correct a deformity. In any case, a "fixed" deformity (a deformity with stiffness) is more disabling. Therefore, hands with deformity should be treated and not neglected.

The aims of treating hands with deformity are:

— to prevent the fingers and thumb becoming stiff;
— to get rid of, or at least prevent further worsening of, any stiffness that is already present.

The following table shows the site of stiffness in the different deformities.

Deformity	Site of stiffness
Claw fingers	Middle joint of fingers
Claw thumb	Tip of thumb
Drop-wrist	Wrist, joints of fingers and thumb

Causes of stiffness

Fingers with deformity become stiff for two reasons:

1. Injury and scarring.
2. Long-standing untreated deformity.

When a joint moves through its full range of movement, the tissues in front and behind the joint (and on the sides if there is also side-to-side movement) become stretched (Fig. 27(a) and (b)). When there is deformity, the joint does not move through its full range, and the tissues on one side remain relaxed and unstretched. Eventually this unstretched tissue becomes shortened (Fig. 27(c)). The shortened tissue does not permit correction of the deformity. The deformity which was previously mobile has now become "fixed", that is, a deformity with stiffness.

Treatment of stiffness

If the tissues on the unstretched side of the joint are kept stretched daily, they will not become shortened and stiffness will not develop. Similarly, if the shortened tissues are gently but firmly stretched daily, continuously

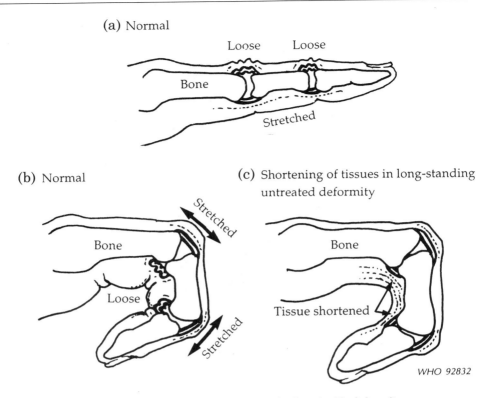

Fig. 27. Shortening of tissues in the hand with deformity

or periodically, they will eventually become longer and stiffness will improve. If the fingers are not stiff, the tissues on the unstretched side can be stretched by exercises. However, if there is some stiffness, these tissues can be stretched and gradually lengthened by massage, and kept stretched by splinting.

Teach patients with deformities of the hand to exercise and massage the fingers and thumbs, as described below. Also splint the fingers, if possible, and teach the patients how to apply splints.

Exercise for the fingers. The patient should keep the knuckles of the fingers firmly bent, using the other hand, as shown in Fig. 28(a). Alternatively, the hand can be pressed against the thigh or the top of a padded bench, table or stool (Fig. 28(c)). Keeping the knuckles bent in this manner, the patient should open the fingers *fully*, until the backs of the fingers touch the other hand or surface (Fig. 28(b) and (d)). This movement should be repeated at least 20 times, twice a day.

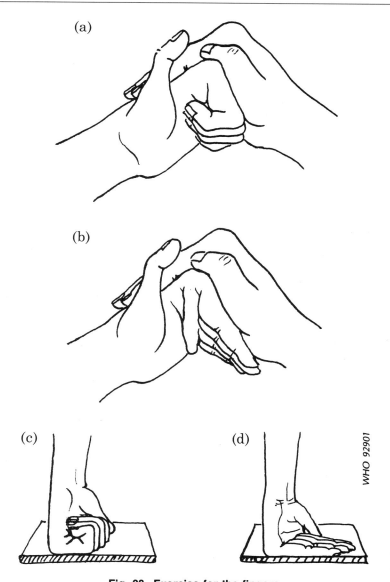

Fig. 28. Exercise for the fingers

Exercise for the thumb. The patient should take hold of the affected thumb with the other hand, steadying it and allowing only the tip of the thumb to move, as shown in Fig. 29(a). Holding the thumb in this manner, the patient should then lift up the tip of the thumb *as much as possible* (Fig. 29(b)). This exercise should be repeated at least 20 times, twice a day.

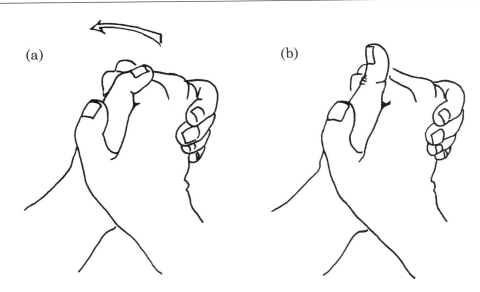

Fig. 29. Exercise for the thumb

Massage for the fingers. The patient should rest the back of the hand on the top of a padded table, bench or stool, or on the thigh (Fig. 30(a)). The patient should then gently stroke the fingers with the other hand, using the edge or the flat of the palm, and straighten them out as much as possible (Fig. 30(b)). Not much force should be used. The patient should do this at least 20 times, twice a day.

Massage for the thumb. The patient should rest the edge of the palm on the top of a padded table, bench or stool, or on the thigh. The patient should then grasp the tip of the thumb with the other hand, as shown in Fig. 31(a) and pull on it gently but firmly, so that the end joint of the thumb

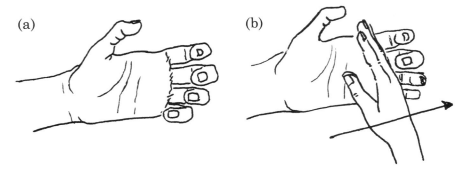

Fig. 30. Massage for the fingers

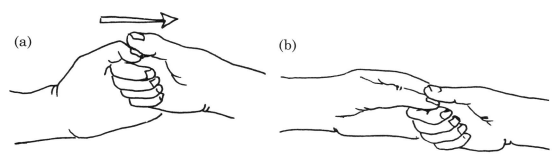

(a)   (b)

Fig. 31. Massage for the thumb

straightens out (Fig. 31(b)). Not much force should be used, otherwise cracks may develop in the skin in front of the end joint of the thumb. The massage should be repeated at least 20 times, twice a day.

In all cases, ensure that the patient has understood the reasons for doing the above exercises and has learnt to do them correctly. Monitor the patient to verify that he or she is practising these exercises and doing them correctly.

Teach the patient to exercise and massage the fingers and thumb at the time of application of oil. Make sure that the patient understands that exercise and massage should not be done when there is a blister or raw area, or when the hand is swollen.

CHAPTER 5

Preventing damage to insensitive feet

This chapter describes the specific actions needed to prevent secondary impairments occurring in feet with impaired sensibility and muscle weakness, and to prevent existing injuries to the feet from worsening.

5.1 Examine to ascertain the risk status

Do a rapid and systematic examination of the feet of all patients at the beginning of the disability prevention programme, and of all new patients thereafter. The aim of this examination is to assess the sensibility of the feet and the condition of the skin, and to detect the presence of muscle weakness, deformity and swelling.

Sensibility testing

Ask the patient whether he or she has normal feeling everywhere in the sole of the foot. Test for perception of pressure with a blunt point (e.g. tip of a ball-point pen), specifically asking whether the patient feels unpleasant pressure or just something touching. Also test for perception of touch, pain and heat, if feasible (see page 24). Test the five sites shown in Fig. 32.

Skin condition

Examine the feet for scars, ulcers, blisters, cracks and wounds.

Deformity

See if there is any shortening or bending or any other deformity of the toes. Check when the patient stands: (i) whether the toes are bent (instead of being straight), and whether the tips of the toes (instead of the pads) are

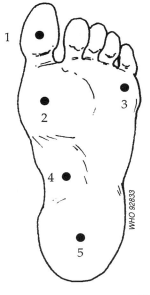

1. Pad of the big toe.
2. Ball of the foot, about 3–4 cm from the crease at the base of the big toe, along a line extending from the midline of the toe.
3. Ball of the foot, about 1.0–1.5 cm from the crease at the base of the little toe, along a line extending from the midline of the toe.
4. Instep.
5. Centre of the heel.

Fig. 32. Sites for testing sensibility

in contact with the ground (Fig. 33(a)); and (ii) whether the sole, including the heel and the big toe side of the ball of the foot, is fully in contact with the ground (Fig. 33(b)).

If the toes are shortened or bent, or if their tips are in contact with the ground during standing, or if any part of the sole other than the instep is not in contact with the ground during standing (Fig. 33(c)), there is deformity in the foot.

Muscle weakness

Ask the patient to walk a few steps and see whether the gait has the normal heel-to-toe pattern (Fig. 34). If you think that the pattern is not normal, ask the patient to take a few steps walking only on the heels (Fig. 35). If the patient cannot do so, this indicates that the leg muscles are weakened.

Swelling

See whether there is any swelling of the toes, foot or ankle. Look below the medial malleolus, which is the bony prominence on the inner (big toe)

(a)

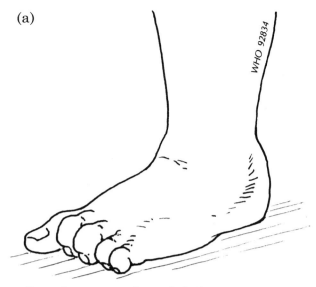

Outer four toes are bent; their tips
(not pads) are in contact with the ground.
This is not normal.

(b)

(c)

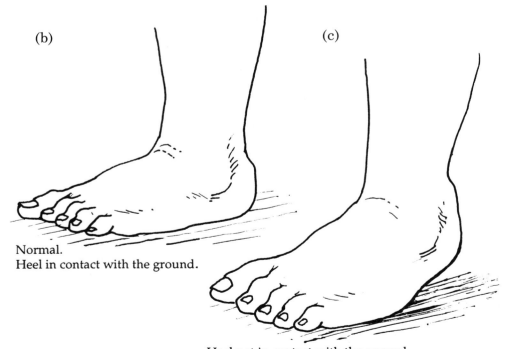

Normal.
Heel in contact with the ground.

Heel not in contact with the ground.
There is a deformity in the foot.

Fig. 33. Shortening or bending of the toes in the foot with deformity

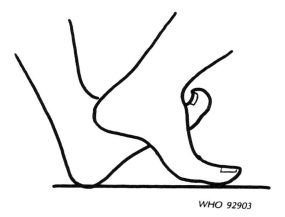

WHO 92903

Fig. 34. Normal heel-to-toe gait

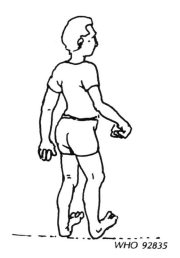

WHO 92835

Fig. 35. Walking on the heels

side of the ankle. Normally there is a shallow depression below this bone Fig. 36(a). When there is swelling of the ankle region, this shallow depression is filled up and the bone is not prominent (Fig. 36(b)).

Feel the foot with the back of your hand to find out whether any area, especially the area where there may be swelling, feels warmer than the surrounding areas, and warmer than the same part in the other foot.

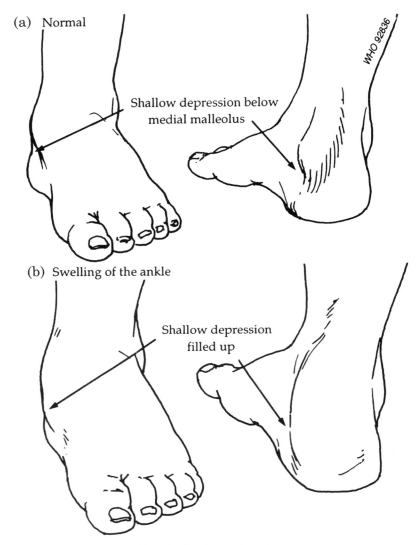

(a) Normal

Shallow depression below
medial malleolus

(b) Swelling of the ankle

Shallow depression
filled up

WHO 92836

Fig. 36. Swelling of the foot

5.2 Assignment of risk status

If any of the following conditions are present, the foot should be categorized as being "in danger": (i) blisters, scars, ulcers, cracks or wounds; (ii) deformity; (iii) muscle weakness; and (iv) swelling.

When there is only loss of sensibility, without any other change, there is a risk of the foot developing an ulcer from external injury. Therefore the foot should be categorized as being "at risk".

If none of the above conditions is present, the foot should be categorized as having "no risk at present". The criteria for determining the risk status are summarized in the following table.

Condition	Risk status and nature of risk
Normal sensibility	No risk at present
Only impaired sensibility (no other abnormality)	"At risk" of injury, ulceration, etc.
Blisters, ulcers, scars, cracks, wounds, deformity, swelling, leg muscle weakness	"In danger" of progressive damage and disability

5.3 Record the risk status of the foot

If the foot is "in danger" or "at risk", this should be recorded prominently in the case chart and the patient register, in order to indicate that further action is required. You may use a special rubber stamp, symbols or colour-coding to indicate the risk status of the foot.

5.4 Assess and record the current impairment status

The degree of impairment should also be recorded in a special disability chart. This record is important as it shows the initial state of the foot and will be needed for future comparison. What you should record and how it is done are shown in the following table.

Condition	Indicate by
Loss or impairment of sensibility	Slanting lines
Scars or callosities	Cross-hatching
Cracks	Lens-like figure
Blisters	"B" enclosed in a circle
Ulcers	Two concentric circles. Indicate size, state (clean or dirty, etc.) and duration
Deformity	"C" for clawing. Indicate degree of clawing, if feasible Indicate level of shortening by " = " sign across the digit
Stiffness	Indicate in writing
Swelling	Indicate in writing
Leg muscle weakness	Indicate strength of muscles in writing or use an arrow ($\downarrow$) to indicate drop-foot

A sample current impairment record for the foot is shown in Fig. 37.

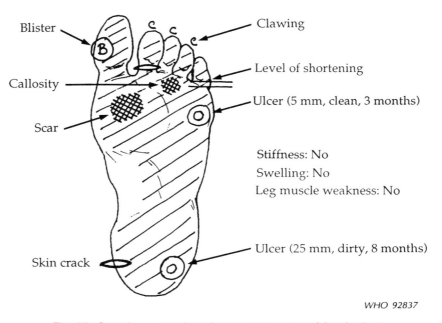

Blister

Clawing

Callosity

Level of shortening

Scar

Ulcer (5 mm, clean, 3 months)

Stiffness: No
Swelling: No
Leg muscle weakness: No

Ulcer (25 mm, dirty, 8 months)

Skin crack

WHO 92837

Fig. 37. Sample current impairment status record for the foot

5.5 Treat treatable conditions

Conditions noted at the time of initial assessment, or at any time later, need to be treated to prevent them worsening. All these conditions can be treated at your level, provided they are identified early. They include:

— scars and callosities
— blisters
— raw areas: cracks, wounds and ulcers
— muscle weakness or paralysis (with or without contractures)
— swelling.

If the above conditions are not treated at an early stage, the foot will get progressively damaged and destroyed and the patient will be crippled.

Priorities

Badly deformed and extensively scarred feet as well as those with long-standing and frequently recurring ulcers are not easy to treat, and the results are not good, even after intensive treatment. The objective of the disability prevention programme is to prevent feet from reaching such a state, not correcting them after they are badly damaged. Therefore, priority should be given to treating the following conditions:

— callosities and thickened skin;
— blisters;
— superficial or uncomplicated raw areas;
— muscle weakness without contractures;
— recent swelling.

Patients with deformities of the feet, long-standing paralysis with contractures, swelling of the foot for more than one month and complicated ulcers will require investigations such as X-rays and medical or surgical treatment as inpatients. Patients with these conditions should be referred to a higher centre for treatment.

Callosities and thickened skin

Common sites

Even normally, the skin of the sole of the foot is thicker than that in other parts of the body. In anaesthetic and non-sweating feet, however, it may become abnormally thick at sites subject to repeated intermittent pressure, especially if footwear is not habitually worn. This abnormally thick skin (called a *callosity* if it is confined to an area) is also more brittle than normal skin and is liable to split and develop *cracks*.

The sites of abnormally thickened skin and cracks commonly seen in anaesthetic feet are shown in Fig. 38. Common sites for thickened skin are: the tips of the toes; the crease between the toes and the ball of the foot; the area under the head of the metatarsal bones; the area under the base of the fifth metatarsal bone near the middle of the outer border of the foot; and the centre and margins of the heel. The sites that commonly develop skin cracks are: the crease between the big toe and the ball of the foot; the area between the pad of the big toe and the ball of the foot; the inner and outer border of the ball of the foot, just below the first and fifth metatarsal bones; and the margins of the heel.

Action required

The objective of treating abnormally thickened skin and callosities is to prevent the skin from developing cracks, by keeping it soft and supple. This is achieved by the daily practice of *skin care* by the patient. Teach the patient skin care and explain why it is important to practise it. Observe the patient to ensure that he or she is practising skin care properly.

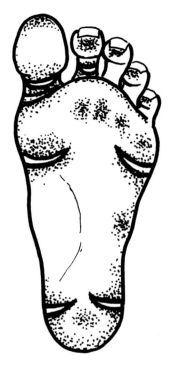

Fig. 38. Common sites for thickening of the skin and skin cracks

Skin care practice

Skin care practice consists of four steps, which are:

— Soaking the foot in water
— Scraping the thickened skin
— Softening the skin with oil
— Shaving off the top layers of thickened skin.

Soaking. Soak the foot in a bucket or tub of soapy or salty water for 15–20 minutes once, or preferably twice, a day. This should be done once in the morning and again in the evening.

When there is a raw area in the foot (e.g. a deep crack, wound or ulcer), add boric acid crystals and calcium hypochlorite (bleaching powder) to the water (2.5 grams of each to 1 litre of water). This will prevent the raw area getting infected and becoming septic.

Scraping. After soaking, scrape the thickened skin with a rough cloth or surface (e.g. a pumice stone). This is to remove the top layers of the thickened skin. Any piece of metal or pottery or a stone with a rough surface may be used for this purpose. Take care not to draw any blood during scraping. Thin the skin in this manner over several days, not all at once. After scraping, wash the foot with water.

Softening the skin with oil. After washing, do *not* dry the skin. Apply some oil (or liquid paraffin) while the foot is wet, and massage it into the skin. The whole foot, including the toes, should be massaged with oil. This helps the skin to retain moisture and will keep it soft and supple.

Shaving. In some cases it may be necessary to shave off the superficial layers of thickened skin (callosities and corns). This should be done using a sharp scalpel, blade or knife, or a sharp pointed stout pair of scissors. Hold the instrument parallel to the skin surface and shave off the superficial layers of thickened skin (Fig. 39(b)). Do not hold the instrument vertically (Fig. 39(a)). In that case you will cut into the foot. As with scraping, there should be no bleeding after shaving.

If the skin is very thick, softening ointment (e.g. salicylic acid, 5% ointment), if available, may be used. The ointment should be applied over the hard skin and rubbed in well, two or three times a day. This will soften the superficial layers and they can then be removed by scraping.

Callosities on toes

Besides the sole of the foot, callosities and corns may develop on the top of the fifth and fourth toes, or on the top and side of the foot near the base of

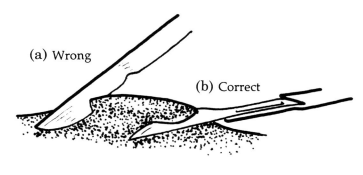

(a) Wrong

(b) Correct

WHO 92904

Fig. 39. Shaving thickened skin

the fifth toe (Fig. 40). This occurs in people who use footwear and indicates that the upper part of the footwear (e.g. straps of sandals or uppers of shoes) is pressing on the top of these toes. This may be because the footwear is too tight (not the correct size) or because the toes are deformed (straps not correctly located). In any case, the pressure on the toes should be relieved. If that is done, the callosity will eventually disappear.

Callosities over the lateral malleolus and the top of the outer part of the foot

Callosities may also develop over the lateral malleolus and the top of the outer part of the foot (Fig. 41). These areas are subjected to high pressure and friction repeatedly in certain sitting positions. These include all those

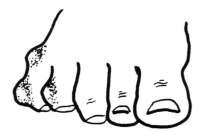

Fig. 40. Callosities on the toes

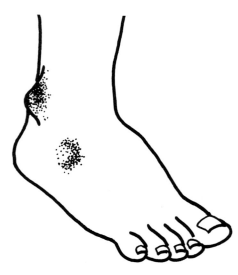

Fig. 41. Callosities over the outer side of the foot and ankle

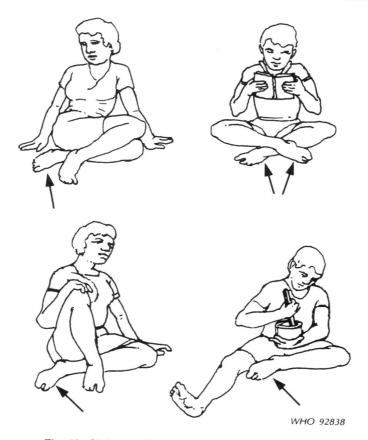

Fig. 42. Sitting positions that give rise to callosities

in which the body rests on the outer surface of the leg and ankle and top of the outer part of the foot. Some of these positions are shown in Fig. 42. Instruct the patient to avoid these positions as much as possible. If the patient has to use any of these positions, instruct the patient to put some soft material (e.g. a pillow or rolled-up cloth) between the ankle and the ground. This will protect the skin over the lateral malleolus and the outer part of the top of the foot. If cracks or wounds etc. develop in these areas, they will not heal easily. Therefore it is very important to prevent them.

Blisters

Causes

Patients tend to assume that all blisters are due to burns. That is not so. Blisters develop in the foot from three causes:

1. Heat (burns)—from contact with hot liquid or a hot surface.
2. Friction—usually from rubbing of straps or edges of footwear, or occasionally from excessive walking or running.
3. Pressure—from walking without appropriate footwear, which causes breakdown of tissue in the sole of the foot, because of repeated high pressure at one particular spot.

When you find a blister, ask the patient what he or she was doing just before the blister appeared, and whether the foot was in contact with hot liquid or a hot surface. Ask for details and try to determine the cause of blistering in order to find a way to prevent repetition of a similar injury.

Action required

Remember that a blister is a wound that is still covered with skin. If the wound is uncovered and gets exposed to infection, it may become septic. Therefore, do *not* break open or puncture the blister. Clean the part well, but gently, without breaking the skin, with soap and water, and mop it dry. Cover the blister with a bulky layer of clean or sterile cloth or gauze, pad it and the surrounding area well with clean cotton wool, and then bandage firmly, preferably with an elastic bandage.

Teach the patient how to bandage firmly, so that he or she can rebandage the affected area when necessary, without disturbing the cotton wool padding. If the blister is between the toes or close to a toe (Fig. 43(a)), put some padding between all the toes so that they are kept apart (Fig. 43(b)). Otherwise, the toes will rub against each other, causing further problems.

(a) (b)

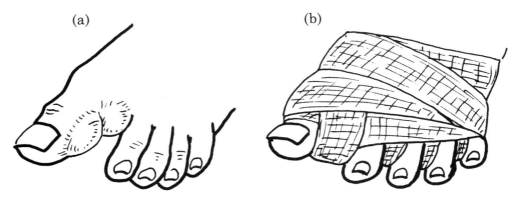

WHO 92905

Fig. 43. Dressing a blister in the front part of the foot

Instruct the patient to rest the foot for at least 72 hours. This is essential when there are blisters on the sole or the toes. The blistered foot should not be put down on the ground, or made to bear weight. The patient should be given a sling and crutches to use during walking, if necessary (see Fig. 44(b)). For blisters caused by burns on the top of the foot, such rest is beneficial, though it might not be essential. Instruct the patient to keep the foot elevated when lying down.

Blister management

- Clean
- Cover
- Pad well
- Bandage firmly
- Rest
- Elevate

If at any stage the blister breaks open, treat it as a raw area (see page 66). Otherwise, instruct the patient to rest the foot as described above and examine it again after 72 hours. If there is increased swelling or redness of the foot, or if the blister has increased in size, refer the patient for further investigation and treatment. If the foot has improved, continue the same line of treatment until the blister completely subsides.

If there is no history of contact with hot liquid or a hot surface and no history of excessive walking or running, the blister is almost certainly due to breakdown of deep tissue because of walking without appropriate footwear. In such cases, the foot should ideally be rested in a plaster cast for three weeks (Fig. 44(a)).

The second best option is for the patient to use a sling for the foot and crutches during walking, so that the affected foot is kept off the ground (Fig. 44(b)).

The third option is to use crutches during walking without the sling (Fig. 44(c)).

The fourth and less satisfactory option is to walk only on the heel of the affected foot when there is a blister or raw area in the front part of the foot (where it is most common), or only on the front part of the foot when there is a blister or raw area in the heel area (which is not common), using a cane or stick for support (Fig. 44(d)).

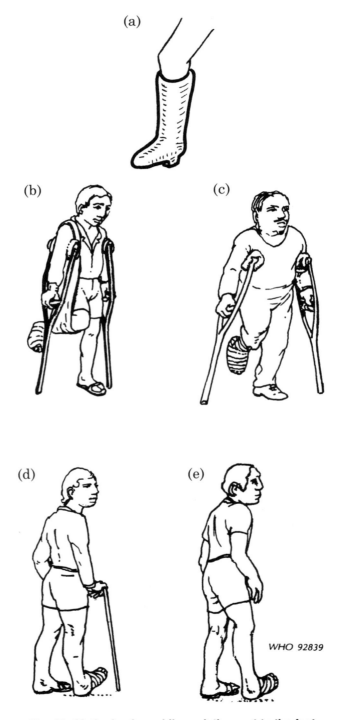

Fig. 44. Methods of providing relative rest to the foot

The fifth and least satisfactory option is to walk with a limp, putting less weight on the affected foot (Fig. 44(e)). However, even this is better than normal walking.

Available options for patients with blisters on the foot caused by walking:

- Resting the foot in a plaster cast
- Using a sling for the foot and crutches during walking
- Using crutches during walking, keeping the foot off the ground
- Walking on the unaffected part of the foot, using a cane or stick
- Limping

In any case, patients who have developed blisters because of high pressures from walking should, as far as possible, avoid putting weight on the affected foot for at least three weeks. After three weeks of resting the foot in this manner, they can use the foot normally, provided that it is protected by special footwear with soft microcellular rubber (or equivalent) insoles.

Raw areas in the foot

Skin cracks, wounds and ulcers in the foot are collectively called "raw areas".

Raw areas may be:

— small or large;
— recent or long-standing (chronic);
— superficial or deep;
— simple or complicated;
— relatively clean or septic and acutely inflamed.

The first three sets of terms are self-explanatory. A raw area is said to be *complicated* when, in addition to the skin, deeper structures such as tendons, bones or joints are involved (Fig. 45). Deep raw areas (e.g. ulcers) are often complicated. When there is only a mild discharge of bloodstained fluid and no discharge of pus, the raw area is said to be *relatively clean*. When there is some discharge of pus, the raw area is *dirty*. When there is much swelling or discharge of foul-smelling pus from one or more sites in the foot, the foot is said to be *septic*. In such cases, there may also be enlarged, tender and painful lymph glands in the groin, fever, and pain in the foot. Patients with septic feet should be referred immediately to an appropriate centre for further investigation and treatment. However,

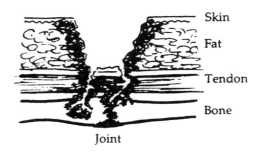

Skin

Fat

Tendon

Bone

Joint

Fig. 45. A deep raw area

patients with relatively clean as well as dirty raw areas can be treated at the peripheral or clinic level.

The principles of management of a raw area are the same, whether the raw area is a crack, wound or an ulcer. They are:

— to *clean* the raw area;
— to *cover* the raw area, to keep it clean; and
— to *rest* the part to permit healing.

The time required for healing varies, depending upon the type of raw area. Wounds usually heal in a few days, while skin cracks take 1–2 weeks and ulcers take 3–6 weeks to heal. Dirty and, especially, septic raw areas also take longer to heal than relatively clean raw areas.

Cleaning

Wash the foot well with soap and water. Scrub the skin of the foot, including the areas between the toes, with a piece of clean cloth or a soft brush to remove all traces of dirt. Do not rub the raw area. Carefully remove any foreign bodies such as sand, gravel or splinters (using a clean pair of forceps) and any other dirt or dead tissue.

Dry the foot well using a clean towel or cloth. Do not rub the raw area, but mop it dry. Do *not* use cotton wool for drying the raw area.

Covering

If the raw area is simple, relatively clean and superficial, it can be covered with strips of ordinary zinc oxide sticking plaster. The strips should be 5–8 mm wide. Apply the plaster strips directly over the raw area, ensuring that each strip overlaps the previous one by 2–3 mm (Fig. 46).

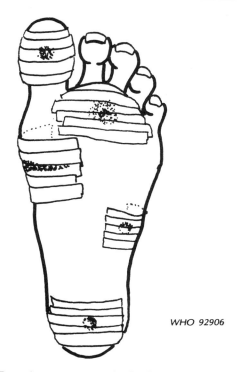

WHO 92906

Fig. 46. Dressing a raw area in the foot using sticking plaster

If sticking plaster is not available, use two layers of clean (sterile, if possible) gauze or cloth to cover the raw area. There is usually no need to apply local medications. However, if you are using a gauze or cloth dressing and there is some discharge from the raw area, the dressing may stick to the raw area. This can be prevented by applying an antiseptic ointment, if available, or using gauze or cloth soaked in sterile petroleum jelly, liquid paraffin or oil. Place a few layers of soft clean cloth or gauze on top of this dressing and cover with a bandage to keep the dressing in place.

If the raw area is deep:

1. Cover it with sticking plaster, gauze or cloth, as described above.
2. On top of it, pack the wound with loosely rolled-up cotton wool, gauze or cloth, so that it fits snugly into the area, without leaving any dead space inside, and the top of the pack is level with the skin surface.
3. Put a second layer of gauze or sticking plaster on top of this pack to keep it in place. If gauze or cloth is used, put a bandage on top of the dressing (Fig. 47).

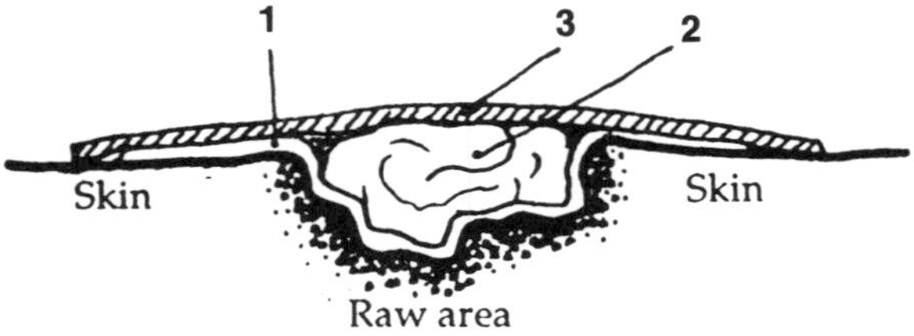

1. Layer of gauze, cloth or sticking plaster.
2. Rolled-up gauze, cloth or cotton wool to fill the depression.
3. Top layer of gauze or sticking plaster.

WHO 92895

Fig. 47. Dressing deeper raw areas

Care of bandage. The aim of covering the raw area is to prevent it from becoming contaminated. This will not be achieved if the bandage gets wet or very dirty, or becomes displaced. Therefore, instruct the patient:

— to avoid wetting the bandage, and to keep the bandaged foot out of water, or protect it with a plastic wrapping;
— to avoid dirtying the bandage, to the extent possible;
— if the bandage becomes displaced, to put it on properly without delay;
— if the bandage gets wet or dirty, to replace the dressing and bandage the foot again.

Sticking plaster is waterproof and, even if it gets wet, water is unlikely to reach the wound. So very strict precautions against wetting are not necessary if the raw area has been dressed with sticking plaster. In fact, if sticking plaster is used, the foot can be washed with soap and water as usual. However, it should be dried promptly afterwards.

Teach the patient and a family member how to dress the wound and apply the sticking plaster or bandage. Supply the patient with some spare dressings, if possible. In any case, *every patient with insensitive feet should always keep a few pieces of clean gauze or cloth, some sticking plaster and two or three bandages.* There is no need to buy ready-made bandages. Old clothing can be torn up to make two or three rolls of bandage (about 10 cm wide).

Dressing a "dirty" raw area. Soak the foot for 10 minutes in water to which boric acid and calcium hypochlorite (bleaching powder) (2.5 grams of each to 1 litre of water) have been added. Wash the foot well with soap and water, removing all traces of dirt. Carefully remove the dead tissue

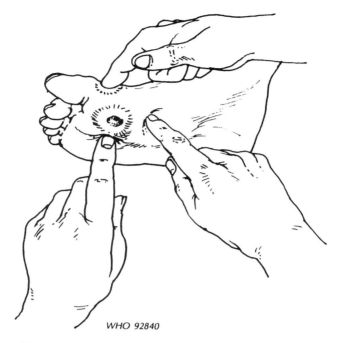

WHO 92840

Fig. 48. Checking the raw area for evidence of infection

and any foreign bodies from the raw area, using clean forceps. Press gently but firmly all around the raw area, the instep region, and the top of the foot to ensure that there are no trapped pockets of pus (Fig. 48).

Dry the foot using a clean towel or cloth. Do *not* rub the raw area, but mop it dry. Do *not* use cotton wool for drying the raw area.

Apply the sticking plaster or other dressing, as described on pages 66–67.

Resting

The raw area will heal by itself, provided it is allowed to do so. If it is subjected to physical stress, healing will be delayed. Therefore, the affected foot must be rested.

Absolute rest. The best way to rest the raw area and protect it from physical stress is to put the patient to bed and keep the foot raised (Fig. 49). However, unless the patient has a septic foot and is ill, absolute rest is not necessary. In most cases relative rest is sufficient.

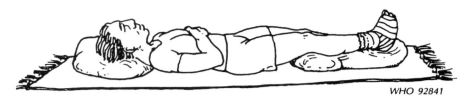

Fig. 49. Absolute rest

Relative rest. Relative rest means that the patient is allowed to move around but takes care to avoid various kinds of physical stress to the raw area. Such kinds of stress are all caused by walking and can be avoided, or at least minimized, in a number of ways, as described on pages 63–65.

How often to dress the raw area

Relatively clean raw areas need not be dressed daily. Instruct the patient to change the dressing every 3–4 days unless it gets wet or the discharge soaks through, in which case it should be changed immediately.

Dirty raw areas may need to be dressed daily (after soaking) until they become relatively clean and the discharge has become minimal.

Muscle weakness in the leg

You should diagnose muscle weakness in the leg when you find that the patient cannot lift the toes or the foot, or cannot keep them lifted up for at least 30 seconds, or cannot stand or walk on the heels. These difficulties indicate that the muscles in the front of the leg are becoming weak or paralysed. Onset of muscle weakness in the leg also shows that the common peroneal nerve on that side is getting damaged. If the patient cannot lift the foot at all, this means that the leg muscles are completely paralysed and the patient has drop-foot (also called foot-drop).

Onset of muscle weakness in the leg suggested by:

- Inability to lift the toes
- Inability to lift the foot
- Inability to keep the toes or foot lifted
- Inability to stand on the heels
- Inability to walk on the heels

Consequences of drop-foot

When there is drop-foot, the patient has to lift the affected leg high during walking (as if he or she is climbing up steps) in order to keep the foot clear of the ground. This makes the person with drop-foot walk with a characteristic high-stepping gait. The joints of the foot are also out of balance, which makes walking and running difficult. The patient cannot run at all when both feet are affected. In addition, paralysis of the leg muscles causes uneven distribution of loads and stresses in the foot during walking and the outer part of the sole of the foot is made to bear more weight than normal. This eventually gives rise to ulceration in the sole, near the base of the little toe or over the outer part of the middle of the foot. Long-standing drop-foot causes the foot to become stiff and twisted. Such deformities, besides making walking difficult, damage the foot badly and cripple the patient.

Drop-foot gives rise to:

● High-stepping gait
● Ulceration
● Unstable foot joints
● Twisted and stiff foot

Therefore, weakness of the leg muscles should be recognized early and treated.

Action required

Onset of leg muscle weakness indicates that the common peroneal nerve is getting damaged and this requires immediate attention to prevent nerve destruction and to promote recovery of the nerve. The patient must be referred to a centre where suitably trained persons will be able to carry out detailed examinations and provide appropriate treatment. You will have to monitor the patient to ensure that the advised treatment is followed. Treatment of this condition is discussed in Chapter 6.

Here, note the following points:

— treatment with anti-leprosy drugs should be started (or continued);
— treatment with prednisolone should be given if necessary;
— the calf muscles should be stretched regularly to prevent shortening;
— when there is acute neuritis of the common peroneal nerve, the knee should be splinted; and

— when there is drop-foot, the patient should use a foot-raising device (see page 74) to permit normal walking.

Check that the patient has understood the need for each aspect of treatment and is following the treatment advice properly.

Patients with leg muscle weakness may need, in addition to anti-leprosy drugs and prednisolone:

- Splinting of knee
- Stretching of calf muscles
- Foot-raising device

Splinting the knee. When there is acute neuritis of the common peroneal nerve and drop-foot, the knee must be splinted to prevent it from bending repeatedly, so that the inflamed nerve is allowed to rest and given a chance to heal quickly. Ready-made splints or plaster slabs are usually available in hospitals or surgical facilities, but not in peripheral areas. You can make a splint, however, using a stiff board or plank about 60 cm long and 10 cm wide. Pad it well, making the central part (which will lie behind the knee) much thicker, lay it behind the knee so that the knee is bent slightly, and bandage it firmly to the leg as shown in Fig. 50.

At night, and whenever the patient is lying down, the foot should be supported to prevent it from dropping down. When there is drop-foot, the weak or paralysed muscles in the front of the leg get pulled and stretched, and that delays their recovery. A simple and easily made splint as shown in Fig. 51 can be used to support the foot. The splint should reach up to the upper part of the thigh and be large enough to support the entire foot. It should be padded well before use.

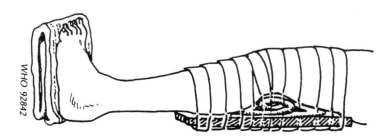

WHO 92842

Fig. 50. Splinting the knee

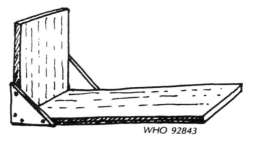

WHO 92843

Fig. 51. A wooden splint

Stretching calf muscles. Muscles are normally kept stretched by various movements. If they are not kept stretched in that manner, they become shorter and contractures (fixed deformities) with stiff bent joints develop. When there is drop-foot, normal stretching of the calf muscles does not occur and, if the condition is neglected, these muscles become shortened, giving rise to permanent raising of the heel. Patients with this deformity have to walk on the front part of the foot, which then gets damaged. All these problems can be prevented by the regular practice of calf-stretching exercises.

The patient stands straight about 60 cm in front of a wall. He or she then leans forward as far as possible, supporting the body with the hands as shown in Fig. 52, *without bending the knees or lifting the heels.* The patient

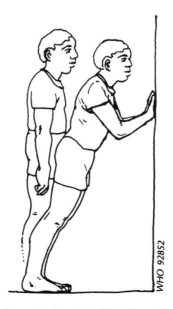

WHO 92852

Fig. 52. Exercise for stretching the calf muscles

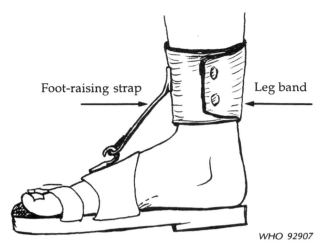

Foot-raising strap   Leg band

WHO 92907

Fig. 53. A foot-raising device

should stay in this position for a full five seconds (a count of five). This exercise should be repeated about 10–15 times, twice a day.

Foot-raising device. Patients with drop-foot need to use special footwear in order to improve their gait and also for even distribution of pressure on the sole. If no such footwear is available or if there is likely to be much delay in obtaining it, a simple foot-raising device can be made and fitted from locally available materials (Fig. 53). Basically, this consists of a leather leg band which fits just above the ankle with a strap, which is attached to the footwear in such a way that the strap holds up the foot and prevents it from dropping. The leg band should be about 10 cm wide and padded, so that it will not damage the skin. The foot-raising strap should be elastic. Rubber (from old tyres) is often used for the foot-raising strap. It should be hooked onto the footwear at a point between the third and fourth toes, on the upper straps of sandals or the uppers of shoes. Use of the foot-raising device will protect the foot and also abolish the high-stepping gait that identifies the person as having drop-foot due to leprosy.

Corrective surgery. Patients who have drop-foot for one year or longer are best treated by corrective surgery, which gives very good results. They should be referred to the nearest centre where such surgery is carried out.

Recent swelling of the foot

Onset of swelling of the foot is a serious condition and must be attended to without delay.

Causes

The causes of swelling of the foot are similar to those for the hand, namely: infection with inflammation (septic foot); injury with inflammation without infection; and inflammation due to reaction. Swelling of both feet is often a sign of a general disorder such as anaemia, heart disease, liver disease or kidney disease. Therefore, patients with this condition should be referred for further investigation and treatment.

Causes of swelling of the foot

Both feet:
- Anaemia
- Heart disease
- Liver disease
- Kidney disease

One foot:
- Infection and inflammation
- Injury and inflammation
- Inflammation due to reaction

The most common cause of swelling of one foot is severe infection and inflammation associated with a plantar ulcer (septic foot). This requires urgent medical and other treatment.

Swelling of the foot due to injury and inflammation is less common; however, this happens more often in the foot than in the hand. For example, a broken bone or a damaged joint may cause inflammation and swelling, which will worsen if the condition is not recognized and treated promptly.

Occasionally, the foot may be involved during reactions and become swollen; however, this occurs less frequently in the foot than in the hand. More often there is bilateral ankle oedema (puffiness or swelling around both ankles) during reactions. Such swelling is not due to infection, injury or inflammation and, except for bandaging the foot firmly and keeping the foot up, it does not require any special treatment.

Action required

First, you must decide why the foot has become swollen. Then, you must take the necessary action, as indicated below.

Swollen foot

- Look for dirty ulcer, recent wounds, recently healed ulcer
- Ask about history of injury
- Feel for warmth

Examine the foot to find out whether there is a dirty or recently healed ulcer, or a recent penetrating wound caused by a thorn, nail or some other sharp object. Also feel the swollen foot with your hands to see whether it is much warmer than the other foot. If so, the foot is most probably septic and the patient will require immediate medical and other treatment (e.g. immobilization of the foot). Refer the patient to the nearest centre where such treatment is available.

If the foot does not appear to be septic, find out whether it has been recently hurt by some injury such as a fall or twisting. If so, there is probably some bone or joint damage and the patient will require further examination and investigation (e.g. an X-ray) and other special treatment. Therefore, refer the patient to the nearest centre where facilities for such investigations and treatment are available.

If there is going to be much delay in getting the patient to such a centre, or if you are not sure about any injury, bandage the foot and keep it up for three days. If the foot has improved by then, continue the treatment for another three days and examine it again. If there has been no marked improvement after 9–15 days, there is probably some serious injury, and you will need to refer the patient immediately for further investigation and treatment. Similarly, if the condition of the foot worsens at any time, this means that it is probably septic and you will have to refer the patient for higher-level medical care. However, if the condition of the foot keeps improving, it is likely that the injury was not a serious one and there is no need to refer the patient.

If there is no history of injury and no evidence of infection, check whether the patient is developing reaction. "Reaction foot" is not at all common and such patients will need to be referred to an appropriate centre for treatment.

If there is no injury or reaction and no obvious evidence of a septic foot (e.g. dirty ulcer, pus under the skin, fever, swelling of the lymph glands in the groin, pain), examine the patient carefully again. Perhaps the patient does not remember an injury or you have missed a septic spot. If you are still in doubt, treat the foot as for injury and examine it again after three days. By that time there will be some definite improvement if the swelling was due to an injury. There will not be much improvement if the swelling was due to infection, and the condition may even have become worse. If it worsens during this time, the foot is most probably septic and you will have to refer the patient immediately to an appropriate centre for treatment.

The above points are summarized in Fig. 54.

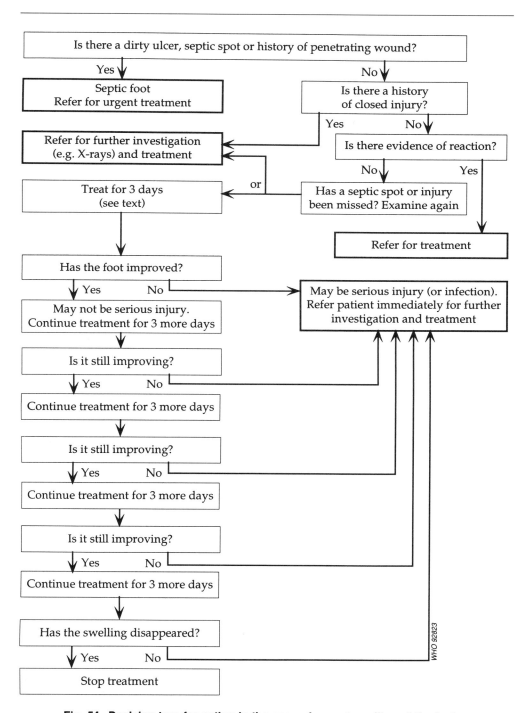

Fig. 54. Decision tree for action in the case of recent swelling of the foot

Treatment

Whatever the cause of swelling of the foot, the causative factor (e.g. infection, injury or reaction) needs to be treated and the foot also requires some special treatment measures. These are: compression bandaging, elevating the foot and resting it in a splint.

Treatment of recent swelling of the foot includes:

- Compression bandaging
- Elevation
- Rest in a splint

Compression bandaging. A pressure bandage providing uniform compression all round the swollen part will help to reduce the swelling in the foot. Use elastic (crepe) bandages if they are available. Keep some of these bandages in two sizes (10 cm and 15 cm width) in stock. If elastic bandages are not available, use strips of ordinary cloth (*not* gauze bandage) for compression bandaging.

Wrap the foot and lower leg with a layer of cotton wool, leaving the toes exposed, and bandage firmly if you are using elastic bandage, or tightly if you are using ordinary cloth bandage. You can get better and more uniform compression if, as you are bandaging, you place a layer of cotton wool over the bandaged area and continue bandaging until you have three alternating layers of cotton wool and bandage. Use figure-of-eight loops while bandaging to provide even compression (Fig. 55).

Elevating the foot and resting it in a splint. A patient who has recently developed a swollen foot should not walk on that foot because a bone in the foot may have been broken or an infection may be developing in the

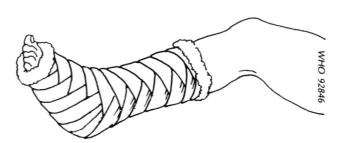

Fig. 55. Compression bandaging

foot. The foot must be rested for it to heal. Elevation, along with compression bandaging, will help to reduce the swelling more quickly. Therefore, the foot should be kept elevated (raised) and rested in a splint. If ready-made splints are not available, a splint can be made from two pieces of wood, as shown in Fig. 56(a) (see page 72). The splint should be padded well before use. The bandaged foot should be secured to the splint with some bandage and kept elevated over some pillows or a box (Fig. 56(b)). It is advisable for you to keep a few such splints in stock. You should also ensure that patients with frequent foot problems have such a splint, or preferably a box splint (Fig. 57), to rest the leg and foot as and when that becomes necessary.

(a)

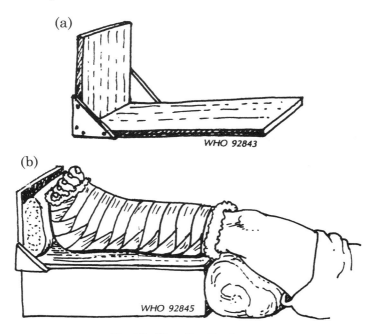

(b)

Fig. 56. Elevating the foot

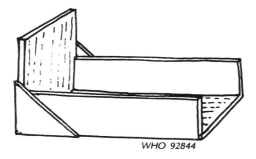

Fig. 57. A box splint

CHAPTER 6

Preserving nerve function

6.1 Recognize damage early

In most leprosy patients, nerve destruction does not occur immediately. It starts as minor damage with minimal loss of function and then progresses to more extensive and more severe loss, ending in complete paralysis of the nerve. Even at that stage, if treated properly, the nerve may recover substantially, if not completely. However, no recovery is possible when the nerve has been destroyed.

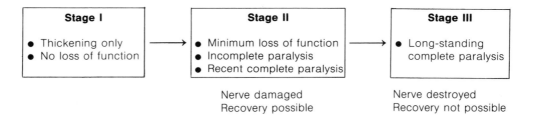

Stage I	Stage II	Stage III
● Thickening only ● No loss of function	● Minimum loss of function ● Incomplete paralysis ● Recent complete paralysis	● Long-standing complete paralysis
	Nerve damaged Recovery possible	Nerve destroyed Recovery not possible

Therefore, if nerve damage is recognized and treated early, the affected nerve will recover in most cases, nerve function will be preserved, and disabilities and deformities will be prevented.

To preserve nerve function

1. Recognize onset or worsening of nerve damage
2. Treat the affected nerve

Recognize onset of nerve damage

When a nerve is in the stage of involvement (see page 6), it is not possible to predict whether it will improve with anti-leprosy treatment or whether it will become damaged and eventually destroyed. The only way to prevent destruction of a nerve trunk is to recognize the onset of nerve damage early and treat it properly.

Recognize onset of nerve damage and treat at that stage

To detect the onset of nerve damage, you need to examine those at risk periodically and systematically for evidence of loss of nerve function, e.g. loss of sweating, impairment of sensibility or sensory loss, and weakness or paralysis of muscles in the hands or feet. In addition, you should instruct and train the patient (and a family member) to recognize the onset of nerve damage (see page 132).

Onset of nerve damage recognized by detecting:

- Areas of loss of sweating
- Areas of sensory loss
- Weakness or paralysis of some muscles in a previously normal part of the hand or foot

Recognize worsening of nerve damage

As with onset, if worsening of nerve damage is recognized early and treated properly, the affected nerve will recover in most cases, and worsening of the impairment(s) will be prevented and severe disability avoided.

Recognize worsening of nerve damage and treat it early

To ascertain whether the damage is progressing in a nerve trunk, you need to examine those affected periodically and systematically for evidence that the loss of function is increasing in extent or severity.

Worsening of nerve damage indicated by:

- Increase in areas of loss of sweating
- Increase in areas of impaired sensibility
- Increase in severity of sensory loss
- Increase in muscle weakness or paralysis

Recognize loss of sweating

Loss of sweating can be seen and the area of such loss can be mapped out without difficulty in countries where people sweat a lot because of the hot and humid climate. In other places this can be difficult to do, especially under field conditions. To find out about loss of sweating in the palms and soles: (i) ask the patient about it; (ii) look at the palms and soles; and (iii) feel them.

Loss of sweating

- Ask the patient about loss of sweating in the palms and soles
- Look at the palms and soles
- Feel the palms and soles for loss of sweating

Ask the patient whether he or she has noticed any areas in the palm or sole that do not sweat and remain dry.

Examine the palms and soles and see if you can identify the areas where sweating does not occur.

Feel the palms and soles of the patient with the back of your hand and determine whether the skin is moist and cool or dry and warmer (or cooler) than other areas. The temperature of non-sweating skin will be closer to that of the surroundings.

If you can make out an area of skin as definitely non-sweating, record this in the patient's chart.

Caution: depending on loss of sweating alone for recognizing onset of nerve damage is not reliable under field conditions; loss of sensibility must be looked for.

Recognize loss of sensibility (sensory loss)

Because of the practical difficulties in reliably diagnosing loss of sweating and because sensory loss occurs well before muscle weakness or paralysis, identifying and mapping out areas of loss of sensibility are necessary to recognize the onset and worsening of nerve damage. To assess loss of sensibility: (i) ask the patient about it; (ii) examine the palms and soles for signs of injury; and (iii) test representative sites in the palms and soles for loss of sensibility (see pages 24 and 50).

> **Sensory nerve damage**
>
> - Ask the patient about loss of sensibility and abnormal sensations
> - Look for wounds, blisters, ulcers and scars
> - Test the palms and soles for perception of pain, heat, touch and pressure
> - Map the areas of sensory loss

Ask the patient whether he or she has any sensory abnormality such as hypersensitive areas, areas with abnormal sensations (e.g. burning, numbness), or areas of dullened sensation. Also ask whether the patient has any areas of loss of sensation, especially that of pain or warmth, in the palms and soles.

Examine the patient's hands and feet for signs of recent or old injuries (e.g. wounds, blisters, ulcers or scars). If present, ask the patient how they occurred, whether pain (or heat) was felt at the time of injury and whether there was any problem with healing. Next, test various sites in the palms and soles (see section 6.2) for loss of pain, heat and touch sensibility using a sharp pin, thermal tester and nylon filament or feather. Lastly, map out the area and type of sensory loss and record any other findings and the date of examination in the patient's chart. This record is an important document as it will be the basis for all future comparisons for detecting the onset or worsening of nerve damage.

While testing for sensory loss, remember the following:

- Pain and heat sensibility are lost earlier than sensibility to light touch. The ability to feel heavy touch, as tested using a blunt point (e.g. the tip of a ball-point pen), is lost very late, and if only heavy touch is tested in the hand, onset of nerve damage will be diagnosed late. Therefore, test for perception of pain and, if possible, heat, for early detection of nerve damage in the hand.
- To the extent possible, carry out the tests in quiet surroundings, to prevent the patient being distracted.
- Test a normal part of the palm and sole to begin with, so that the patient understands what is required of him or her and knows what to expect.
- Do not test just once only. Repeat the testing at least three or four times.
- Do not test the same site continuously.
- Include one or two fake tests, e.g. ask what the patient felt even though you had not done anything.
- Make sure that the patient cannot see what you are doing while testing.

Recognize muscle weakness

Muscle weakness and paralysis usually develop some time after sensory loss and are not an early sign of nerve damage. However, muscle weakness is the cause of paralytic deformities such as claw hand and drop-foot, and by recognizing muscle weakness early and treating it properly at that stage, paralytic deformities can be prevented. While detailed muscle testing (testing and grading the strength of all muscles individually) may not be possible in the field, there are some tests that can be carried out easily and quickly and will help to recognize weakness of certain muscles. Such tests can be used for screening patients for nerve damage and for monitoring their response to treatment. The field worker's diagnosis of muscle weakness must be verified by a senior health worker who will also carry out detailed muscle testing and record the findings for future use.

Ask the patient whether he or she experiences any difficulties in using the hands or in walking, and if so, the nature of the difficulty. Examine the patient's hands, legs and feet for any deformity or other signs of muscle weakness, paralysis or wasting. These signs are described in the next section. Next, carry out one or two tests on each nerve trunk to ascertain whether any muscles supplied by that nerve trunk are weakened or paralysed. These tests are also described in the following section. Record the findings (both normal and abnormal) and the date of examination.

Muscle weakness

- Ask about difficulties in using the hands or in walking
- Look for deformity and other signs of muscle weakness, paralysis or wasting
- Carry out several tests on each nerve trunk
- Record normal and abnormal findings

6.2 Recognize damaged nerve trunks

As mentioned in section 2.3, the nerve trunks that are most commonly damaged and destroyed in leprosy are the ulnar nerve, posterior tibial nerve, median nerve and common peroneal nerve. The radial and facial nerves are only occasionally seriously damaged. However, it is not enough to know that there is nerve damage — you must know which nerve trunk has been affected and to what extent.

As discussed on page 8, nerve trunks are "mixed nerves", that is, they supply an area of skin and a set of muscles. Therefore, by identifying the area of sensory loss (and dry skin) and the muscles that have become weak or paralysed, you can find out which nerve trunk has been damaged.

Identify damaged nerve trunk by:

- Site of loss of sensibility
- Type of muscle weakness

Recognize ulnar nerve damage

Site of sensory loss

The area of loss of sensibility in the palm in the case of ulnar nerve damage is shown in Fig. 58.

Ask the patient about sensory loss or abnormal sensations in this area.

Look for injuries, scars, blisters, ulcers, cracks and dryness in this area.

Feel for dryness of the skin in this area.

Test for loss of sensibility to pain, heat and light touch at two sites (Fig. 59): (i) in the palm, 3–4 cm from the crease at the base of the little finger, along a line extending from the midline of that finger; and (ii) in the pulp of the little finger.

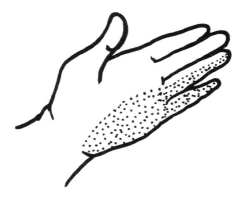

Fig. 58. Site of sensory loss in the case of ulnar nerve damage

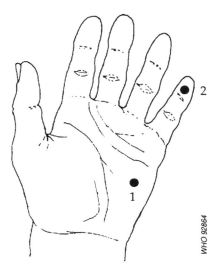

1. Palm, about 3–4 cm from the crease at the base of the little finger, along a line extending from the midline of the finger.
2. Pulp of the little finger.

Fig. 59. Testing for loss of sensibility due to ulnar nerve damage

Muscle weakness

Even complete paralysis of all the muscles supplied by the ulnar nerve does not disable a person very much. Nevertheless, a person with ulnar nerve damage may complain of "weakness of grip", "clumsiness in the use of the hand" or that "the little finger does not cooperate with the others". Therefore:

Ask the patient about any problems in using the hand.

Look for wasting (loss of bulk) of the muscles as evidenced by flattening and straightening of the little finger side of the palm and flattening of the soft bulge of the muscle in the back of the hand between the thumb and the index finger (Fig. 60). Also look for deformity, as evidenced by mild clawing of the little finger.

Test:

1. The patient's ability to keep all the fingers straight and together. In the early stages of ulnar nerve paralysis, the little finger cannot be kept straight and together with the other fingers, and it stays a little apart from the ring finger (Fig. 61(a)). It may also be slightly bent or clawed (Fig. 61(b)).

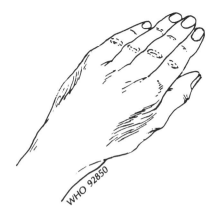

Fig. 60. Sites of muscle wasting due to paralysis of the ulnar nerve

(a)   (b)   (c)

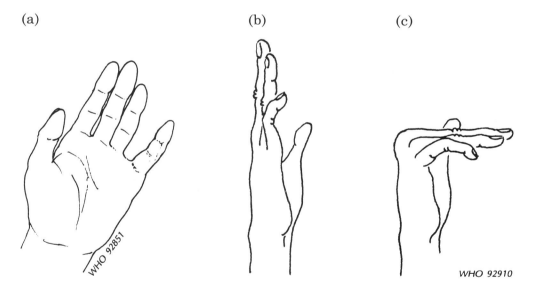

Fig. 61. Testing for muscle weakness due to paralysis of the ulnar nerve

2. The patient's ability to bend all the fingers at the base, keeping the other joints straight, and to keep them like that for about 30 seconds. In early ulnar nerve paralysis, the little finger cannot be kept in this position and it will be bent (Fig. 61(c)).

Record the findings regarding: abnormal sensations, sensory loss and information about muscle wasting, deformity and weakness.

Recognize median nerve damage

Site of sensory loss

The area of loss of sensibility in the palm in the case of median nerve damage is shown in Fig. 62.

Ask the patient about sensory loss or abnormal sensations in this area.

Look for injuries, scars, blisters, ulcers, cracks, wounds and dryness in this area.

Feel for dryness of the skin in this area.

Test for loss of sensibility to pain, heat and light touch at three sites (Fig. 63): (i) in the palm over the thenar eminence, about 1.0–1.5 cm from the crease at the base of the thumb and along a line extending from the midline of the thumb; (ii) in the pulp of the thumb; and (iii) in the pulp of the index finger.

Muscle weakness

Damage to the median nerve causes weakness and paralysis of the muscles that form the bulge at the base of the thumb (thenar eminence). When these muscles become weak or paralysed, they atrophy and the thenar eminence becomes flattened. This causes considerable disability because the thumb is weakened. Holding and manipulating objects become difficult or even impossible.

Ask the patient whether he or she has any difficulty in picking up and holding small objects.

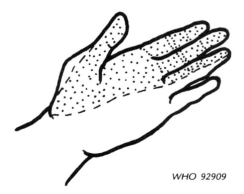

WHO 92909

Fig. 62. Site of sensory loss in the case of median nerve damage

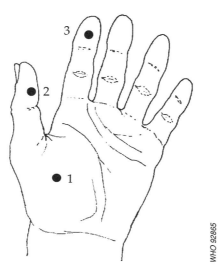

1. Thenar eminence, about 1.0–1.5 cm from the crease at the base of the thumb, along a line extending from the midline of the thumb.
2. Pulp of the thumb.
3. Pulp of the index finger.

Fig. 63. Testing for loss of sensibility due to median nerve damage

Look for wasting or flattening of the thenar eminence. Also look for the deformity of claw thumb, in which the thumb is bent backwards at the wrist and forwards in the middle and at the tip (Fig. 64).

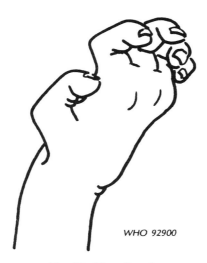

WHO 92900

Fig. 64. Claw thumb

Test the patient's ability to move the thumb away from the palm in a plane perpendicular to it. This can be done in two ways:

1. Ask the patient to stretch the hand out, with the palm horizontal and facing upwards and the fingers and thumb facing forwards. Then ask the patient to lift the thumb upwards (Fig. 65(a)) and hold it in that position for at least 30 seconds. The tip of the thumb should be pointing upwards and not forwards. When the median nerve is damaged, the patient will be unable to hold the thumb in this position.

2. Ask the patient to hold the arms close to the sides of the body with the elbows bent, forearms pointing forwards, fingers and thumbs straight and palms facing each other. Now ask the patient to move the thumbs away from the palms and towards each other, and to hold them in that position for at least 30 seconds (Fig. 65(b)). In the case of median nerve damage, the affected thumb cannot be held sufficiently away from the palm to point towards the other thumb, as shown in Fig. 65(b).

(a)

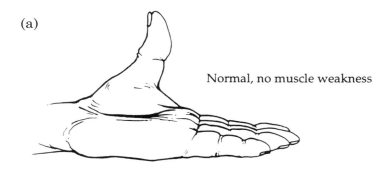

Normal, no muscle weakness

(b)

Weakness of the thumb muscles

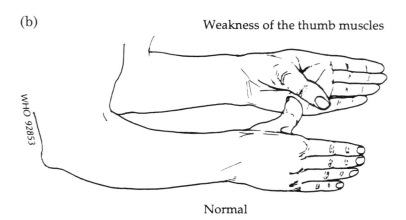

WHO 92853

Normal

Fig. 65. Testing for muscle weakness due to median nerve damage

Record the findings regarding: abnormal sensations, sensory loss, and information about muscle wasting, deformity and weakness.

Recognize damage to the posterior tibial nerve

Site of sensory loss

The areas of loss of sensibility in the case of damage to the posterior tibial nerve or its branches are shown in Fig. 66. While the nerve trunk supplies the entire sole of the foot, its main terminal divisions (the medial and lateral plantar nerves) supply the front and middle parts of the sole, whereas the heel is supplied by the calcaneal nerve, which branches off the nerve trunk at a higher level. In the early stages of damage to the posterior tibial nerve, only a part of the sole may therefore be affected.

Ask the patient about sensory loss or abnormal sensations in these areas.

Look for injuries, scars, blisters, ulcers and cracks in the sole. Also look for sweating in the three parts of the sole.

Feel for sweating in the three parts.

Testing for loss of sensibility in the sole is not easy, because the skin is normally very thick and it becomes even more thickened in people who do

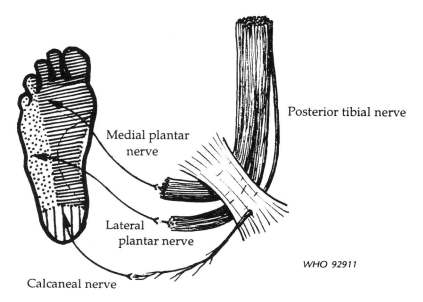

Fig. 66. **Site of sensory loss in the case of damage to the posterior tibial nerve**

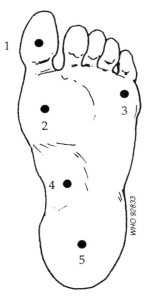

1. Pad of the big toe.
2. Ball of the foot, about 3–4 cm from the crease at the base of the big toe, along a line extending from the midline of the toe.
3. Ball of the foot, about 1.0–1.5 cm from the crease at the base of the little toe, along a line extending from the midline of the toe.
4. Instep.
5. Centre of the heel.

Fig. 67. Testing for loss of sensibility due to damage to the posterior tibial nerve

not habitually wear footwear. Therefore it is not reliable to test for sensibility to heat or light touch in the sole. It is also not possible to test for perception of pain with a sharp pin. However, perception of pressure and pain from deep pressure should be tested, using a blunt point (such as the tip of a ball-point pen). Test the five standard sites shown in Fig. 67.

Muscle weakness

The patient does not experience any noticeable disability from paralysis of the muscles in the sole of the foot supplied by the medial and lateral plantar nerves.

Look for clawing of the toes, which occurs when the posterior tibial nerve is damaged and the muscles in the foot are weakened or paralysed. Instead of being straight (Fig. 68(a)), the toes become curled (clawed), so that the tips of the toes, not their pads, touch the ground (Fig. 68(b)). However, this is not a very reliable indicator of weakness of the muscles in the foot as people who have been habitually wearing shoes often have bent toes.

Testing for weakness or paralysis of muscles in the foot is also difficult and requires some practice. You must practise the following tests on yourself

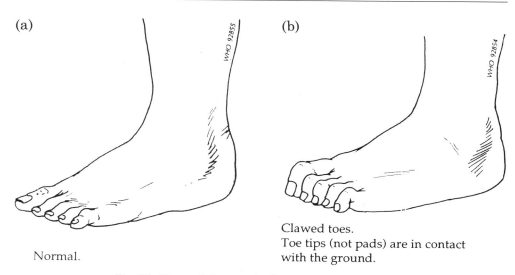

(a) Normal.

(b) Clawed toes.
Toe tips (not pads) are in contact
with the ground.

Fig. 68. Signs of damage to the posterior tibial nerve

so that you can demonstrate them to the patient. The patient should also practise the test a few times on the normal foot.

1. Ask the patient to place the foot firmly on the ground and to press the ground with the big toe, keeping it straight while lifting the other toes (Fig. 69(a)). If the muscles in the foot are weak or paralysed, the big toe will be seen to bend as shown in Fig. 69(b) and you can confirm this by feeling it.

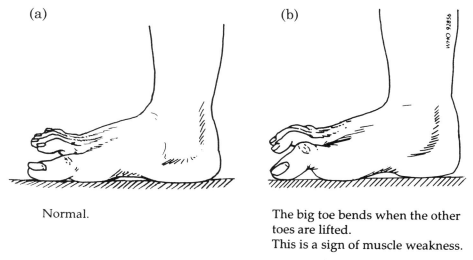

(a) Normal.

(b) The big toe bends when the other toes are lifted.
This is a sign of muscle weakness.

Fig. 69. Testing for muscle weakness due to paralysis of the posterior tibial nerve
1. Press the ground with the big toe, keeping it straight while lifting the other toes

2. Ask the patient to place the foot firmly on the ground, lift all the toes, and spread them out (Fig. 70). While the patient is doing this, watch also for the little toe moving outward. If the muscles in the foot are weak or paralysed, the toes cannot be spread out. However, this is not a very reliable test as people who have been habitually wearing shoes often cannot spread their toes.

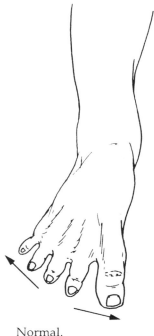

Normal.
All the toes are spread out.

Fig. 70. Testing for muscle weakness due to paralysis of the posterior tibial nerve
2. Spread out all the toes

3. Ask the patient to place the foot firmly on the ground with all the toes touching the ground. Now, ask the patient to draw back or "retract" the toes without lifting them off the ground. Normally such retraction of the toes will be possible by bending the toes like an "S" and the toe pads will be in contact with the ground (Fig. 71(a)). If the muscles of the foot are weak or paralysed, this is not possible. In that case, the toes will be curled like a "C" and the tips of the toes, not the pads, will be in contact with the ground (Fig. 71(b)).

(a) (b)

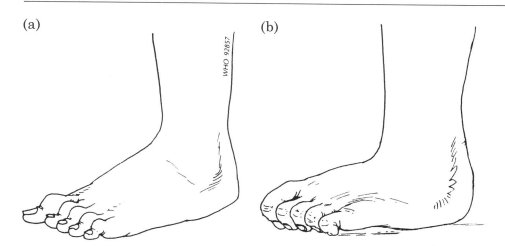

WHO 92857

Normal.
Toes are bent like an "S"; their pads
are in contact with the ground.

Toes are curled like a "C"; their tips
(not pads) are in contact with the ground.
This is a sign of muscle weakness.

**Fig. 71. Testing for muscle weakness due to paralysis of the posterior tibial nerve
3. Retract the toes**

Record the results of each of the above tests as "normal" or "paralysed".
Record the other findings also.

Recognize damage to the common peroneal nerve

Site of sensory loss

The common peroneal nerve supplies a large area of skin on the front of
the leg and top of the foot through its terminal division, the superficial
peroneal nerve. Because the cutaneous branches of this nerve are very
frequently affected in leprosy, sensory loss in the area of supply of the
common peroneal nerve does not necessarily indicate damage to the nerve
trunk. So weakness or paralysis of the muscles supplied by the common
peroneal nerve must be looked for.

Muscle weakness

The common peroneal nerve supplies the bulky muscles in the front of the
leg that lift the foot and toes up, and the muscles on the outer side of the
leg that turn the foot outward. Until these muscles (and so the nerve) are
almost completely paralysed, however, the patient may not have noticed
any disability during walking.

Ask the patient whether he or she has any problem walking and, if so, the nature of the problem. During the early stages of damage to the common peroneal nerve, the muscle that holds the big toe up becomes weak and the patient may find that the big toe "gets in the way" during walking. The patient may also have difficulty in running.

Look at the gait. Ask the patient to walk a few steps and watch the gait. When the muscles in the front of the leg are weak or paralysed, the patient has to lift the affected leg high up when walking, as if he or she is climbing up steps, so as to keep the foot clear of the ground.

Look at the front of the leg for evidence of muscle wasting. Normally, these muscles bulge out in the upper part of the front of the leg. When the common peroneal nerve is damaged, these muscles atrophy and the bulge flattens out, and the shin bone (tibia) becomes prominent.

Carry out the following tests:

1. Ask the patient to take three or four steps walking on the heels, holding the front part of the foot up (Fig. 72(a)). When the muscles in the front of the leg are weak or paralysed, this will not be possible.
2. Ask the patient to put the foot firmly on the ground and lift all the toes, keeping them straight and without lifting the foot. The toes should be held in that position for at least 30 seconds (Fig. 72(b)). Normally the tendons on the top of the foot stand out when the toes are lifted. When the muscles in the front of the leg are weak or paralysed, the patient will not be able to lift his or her toes and the tendons will not stand out.

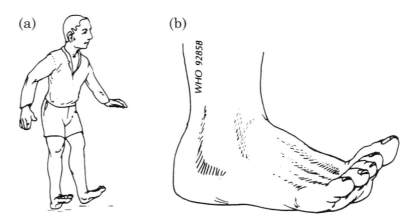

(a)   (b)

WHO 92858

Fig. 72. Testing for muscle weakness due to damage to the common peroneal nerve

3. Ask the patient to sit on a high stool, with both legs dangling, and then lift only the foot, without raising the leg. Alternatively, ask the patient to stand on one leg (holding on to a wall or table for balance) and then lift the foot of the other leg. When the common peroneal nerve is damaged, lifting the foot becomes difficult or impossible.

Record the findings of each of the above tests as normal, weak or paralysed.

Recognize damage to the radial nerve trunk

Site of sensory loss

The radial nerve has two parts, the main or deep radial nerve trunk in the arm, which supplies the muscles in the back of the forearm, and the superficial radial nerve, which supplies the skin on the back of the hand. The superficial radial nerve is very commonly affected in leprosy patients, but the main nerve trunk is only occasionally damaged. Damage to the radial nerve trunk causes severe disability because the wrist and all the joints of the fingers and thumbs are thrown out of balance. However, the nerve trunk usually recovers very well if it is treated early. Therefore it is very important to recognize damage to the radial nerve trunk at an early stage and treat it properly.

As with the common peroneal nerve, sensory loss in the area of supply does not necessarily indicate damage to the radial nerve trunk, because of the very common involvement of the superficial radial nerve in leprosy. You must therefore look for muscle weakness caused by damage to the radial nerve trunk.

Muscle weakness

The radial nerve trunk supplies the muscles (extensors) in the back of the forearm that lift up the wrist, fingers and thumb. When this nerve trunk is damaged, these muscles become weak and the wrist, fingers and thumb cannot be held up.

Ask the patient about problems in using the hand. When extensor muscles are paralysed, it is almost impossible to use the hand.

Look at the muscles in the back of the forearm. When the radial nerve trunk is paralysed, these muscles atrophy.

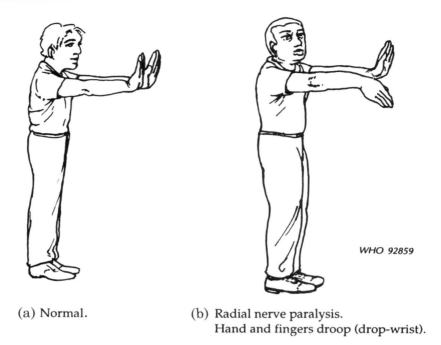

WHO 92859

(a) Normal.

(b) Radial nerve paralysis.
Hand and fingers droop (drop-wrist).

Fig. 73. Testing for muscle weakness due to radial nerve paralysis

Carry out the following test:

Ask the patient to stretch both arms straight in front, holding the hands and fingers up as much as possible, and to keep holding them like that for at least 30 seconds (Fig. 73(a)). When the muscles in the back of the forearm are weak or paralysed, the hand and fingers cannot be held up and on the affected side they will droop down (Fig. 73(b)).

Record the findings of the above test as normal, weak or paralysed.

Recognize facial nerve damage

The facial nerve is also occasionally damaged in leprosy. When that occurs several muscles, including those that move the eyelids, become weak and, if left untreated, this can lead to serious consequences such as ulceration in the eye, loss of vision and loss of the eye. However, like the radial nerve, the facial nerve responds very well to treatment. It is therefore very important to recognize damage to the facial nerve early and to treat it properly.

Site of sensory loss

Each facial nerve supplies only the muscles that move the face on that side. It does not supply the skin. Therefore there is no sensory loss when the nerve is damaged.

Muscle weakness

When the facial nerve is damaged, the muscles in the upper part of the face that move the eyelids and the skin on the forehead become weak. Sometimes all the muscles on one side of the face become weak or paralysed and cause a deformity of the face.

Ask the patient whether he or she has any problems with the eyes. When the eyelid muscles are weak or paralysed, there may be watering of the eye and redness and it will not be possible to close the eye.

Look at the patient's face. The eye on the affected side does not blink as often as that on the normal side and it may be opened wider. There may also be more tears and watering of the affected eye.

When the facial nerve is completely paralysed, the affected side of the face is flattened out, without any folds in the skin and the mouth is pulled towards the normal side by the muscles on that side (Fig. 74).

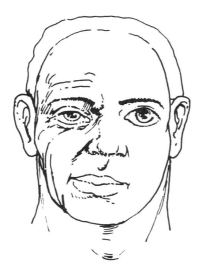

Fig. 74. Signs of paralysis of the facial nerve

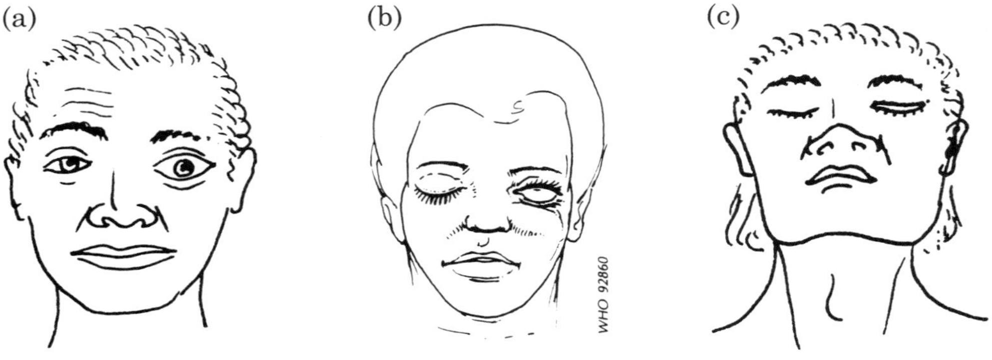

(a)   (b)   (c)

WHO 92860

Fig. 75. Testing for muscle weakness due to paralysis of the facial nerve

Carry out the following tests:

1. Ask the patient to raise the eyebrows, wrinkling the forehead in the process. When the facial nerve is damaged, the eyebrow on the affected side does not go up and the forehead on that side remains flattened and does not become wrinkled (Fig. 75(a)).
2. Ask the patient to close both eyes as tightly as possible and to keep them closed like that for at least 30 seconds. When the eyelid muscles are paralysed, the patient cannot close the eye on that side. Consequently, the eyeball rolls up while the eye remains partly open (Fig. 75(b)). However, when these muscles are weak but not paralysed, the patient usually manages to close the eye by pushing the cheek up on that side of the face.
3. Ask the patient to tilt the chin up and gently close the eyes. When the facial nerve is damaged, the eye on the affected side does not close completely and there is a thin gap between the lids (Fig. 75(c)). This is usually one of the first signs of facial nerve damage.

Record the findings of each of the above tests as normal, weak or paralysed.

6.3 Onset and worsening of nerve damage

Onset of nerve damage

Nerve damage may come on suddenly over a short period of time (acute onset), or it may come on so gradually that the patient may not be aware of anything wrong until the paralysis is almost complete (insidious onset).

Nerve damage of acute onset

This happens quite often during an attack of acute neuritis. During acute neuritis, the nerve trunk becomes swollen, very painful and very tender and the nerve may get damaged within a short time. Attacks of acute neuritis increase the chances of nerve damage very considerably.

Acute neuritis → Nerve damage of acute onset

Nerve damage of insidious onset

Nerve damage of insidious onset is also quite common. It is sometimes known as "quiet nerve paralysis" (QNP), because the affected nerve becomes paralysed "quietly", with no obvious signs and symptoms such as increased tenderness or pain. Because the damage sets in so gradually, the patient may not be aware of loss of sensibility or its extent.

Nerve damage of insidious onset or quiet nerve paralysis
Patient may not be aware of loss of function

Worsening of nerve damage

Nerve damage may worsen irregularly, in bouts, when the nerve is subject to attacks of acute neuritis, the damage increasing with each attack

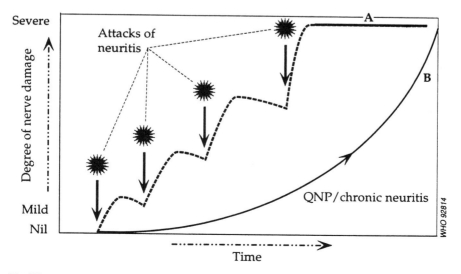

Fig. 76. Worsening of nerve damage in acute and chronic neuritis or quiet nerve paralysis

without much worsening between attacks (A in Fig. 76). On the other hand, nerve damage may worsen continuously and gradually. This occurs in quiet nerve paralysis, in which the nerve may become completely paralysed over the course of many months (B in Fig. 76). Continuous worsening of nerve damage also occurs in chronic neuritis.

6.4 Preserving nerve function

Actions required

The following actions are required to preserve nerve function and prevent nerve damage:

1. The patients at risk of nerve damage must be identified early.
2. Baseline records of the state of the affected and other nerve trunks must be kept and assessed periodically so that onset or worsening of nerve damage is recognized without delay.
3. Patients identified as having nerve damage must be referred for confirmation of the same and for more detailed assessment of nerve function and treatment.
4. Patients must be instructed and trained to recognize and report loss of nerve function and acute neuritis without delay.

To preserve nerve function

1. Identify patients at risk of nerve damage
2. Maintain records of the state of the patients' nerve trunks and assess them periodically
3. Refer patients with nerve damage for further investigation and treatment
4. Instruct and train patients to recognize and report onset or worsening of nerve damage without delay

---

Assess and record the risk status of the nerve trunks

As for the hands and feet, the risk status of each nerve trunk must be assessed and recorded prominently in the case chart and the patient register. The risk status should be classified as "low risk", "at risk" and "in danger of destruction".

Risk status for nerve damage

- Low risk of nerve damage
- At risk of nerve damage
- In danger of destruction

Low-risk nerves

When a nerve trunk is apparently normal, not thickened or tender, it is classified as being at "low risk" of nerve damage. You may use the symbol "√" to indicate low-risk status. Low-risk nerves need not be assessed for damage unless there are signs and symptoms of sensory loss relating to their area of supply. However, the risk status of these nerves must be confirmed periodically, since it may change.

> **Low risk of damage√**
>
> ● Nerve trunk not thickened or tender
> ● No symptoms or signs of sensory loss

"At-risk" nerves

When a nerve trunk is thickened or tender, but as yet there is no evidence of damage, it is classified as being "at risk" of nerve damage. You may use the symbol "?" to indicate "at-risk" status. Nerves at risk of damage must be assessed periodically for evidence of onset of damage.

> **At risk of damage?**
>
> ● Nerve trunk thickened or tender
> ● No evidence of damage

Nerves "in danger" of destruction

When a nerve trunk already shows evidence of some damage, it is "in danger" of destruction. The symbol "!!" may be used to indicate "in danger" risk status. Nerves in the state of acute neuritis should also be classified as in danger of destruction, even when there is no evidence of damage. The nerve trunks of patients with borderline types (in particular, mid-borderline (BB) and borderline tuberculoid (BT)) of leprosy are also classified in this group, because these patients are prone to develop reversal reactions during acute neuritis, which may damage nerves rapidly and severely.

> **In danger of destruction!!**
>
> ● Nerves already showing some damage
> ● Nerves in acute neuritis
> ● Nerves in patients with borderline leprosy

Nerves that are completely paralysed may be considered to be irreversibly damaged and so destroyed, provided that complete paralysis (not onset of paralysis) has been present for at least one year. The symbol "+" may be used to indicate that a nerve trunk has been destroyed. The question of preserving or restoring their function does not arise in these cases. However, actions to prevent worsening of disability will need to be taken.

The decision tree in Fig. 77 shows how the risk status of nerve trunks should be determined.

Using the decision tree, assess the risk status of each nerve trunk and record the results on the case chart and patient register. The risk status of the nerve trunks must be recorded prominently on the patient's records, preferably on the outside cover, using a distinctive colour, code or symbol. The results of follow-up examinations should also be recorded in the same place. A sample record form is shown below.

Nerve trunk	Left side								Right side							
	Initial assessment	Follow-up							Initial assessment	Follow-up						
		1	2	3	4	5	6			1	2	3	4	5	6	
Ulnar	+								?							
Median	✓								✓							
Common peroneal	✓								✓							
Posterior tibial	!!								✓							
Radial	✓								✓							
Facial	✓								✓							
Date of assessment	5.8.92								5.8.92							

The record shows that, at the initial assessment:

— the left ulnar nerve has been destroyed;
— the right ulnar nerve is "at risk" (thickened, but not yet damaged);
— the left posterior tibial nerve is "in danger" of being destroyed (already damaged);
— the other nerves examined were not thickened, tender or painful and so are at "low risk" of damage.

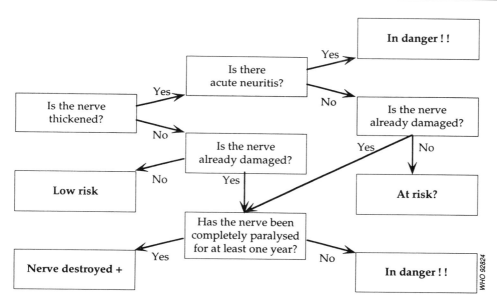

Fig. 77. Decision tree for determining the risk status of nerve trunks

The results of the follow-up examinations should be added to the table as these assessments are done. The risk status may also be recorded using the degree of nerve involvement to indicate the extent of damage in each nerve trunk (see below).

Assess and record the degree of nerve involvement

Having assessed and recorded the risk status for each nerve trunk, the next step is to assess and record the degree of nerve involvement for each nerve trunk. The following grading of the degree of involvement is suggested for this purpose.

Grade/degree of nerve involvement	Criteria
0	No abnormality
1	Thickening, tenderness and pain present; no loss of function
2	Loss of function; incomplete sensory loss
3	Complete sensory loss; no muscle weakness
4	Sensory loss and muscle weakness present, but one or both incomplete
5	Complete sensory loss and muscle paralysis present for less than 12 months
6	Complete sensory loss and muscle paralysis present for at least 12 months

For each nerve trunk, assess and record the degree of its involvement, or get the information from the records of detailed assessment. Do the same for follow-up assessments as well. A sample record form of the degree of nerve involvement is shown below.

Nerve trunk	Left side								Right side							
	Initial assessment	Follow-up							Initial assessment	Follow-up						
		1	2	3	4	5	6			1	2	3	4	5	6	
Ulnar	6								1							
Median	0								0							
Common peroneal	0								0							
Posterior tibial	5								0							
Radial	0								0							
Facial	0								0							
Date of assessment	5.8.92								5.8.92							

Nerves at low risk of damage

These are the apparently normal nerve trunks that are not thickened, tender, painful or damaged (nerve involvement Grade 0). The risk of these nerves becoming damaged is low. They do not therefore require any special attention, except for periodic checking during each clinical assessment or at least once a year during the period of surveillance.

Low-risk nerves

Periodically examine for thickening, tenderness and damage

Nerves at risk of damage

These are the nerve trunks that are thickened (and usually also somewhat tender or painful) but do not as yet show any loss of function, indicating that they have not yet been damaged to any significant extent (nerve involvement Grade 1). As it is not possible to predict whether nerve trunks in this grade will eventually become damaged or destroyed, besides treating leprosy and periodically checking for signs of onset of nerve damage, there is no special action that can be taken. These nerves must be assessed at every clinical assessment, or at least once every 6 months during the period of surveillance. Furthermore, the patient must be trained to check periodically for onset of nerve damage and report immediately if that happens.

At-risk nerves

- Periodically examine for onset of nerve damage
- Train patient to check for nerve damage

Nerves in danger of destruction

These are the nerve trunks that show evidence of reversible nerve damage (nerve involvement Grade 2– 5). In these cases, record the degree of nerve involvement according to the criteria given on page 105. These patients require treatment, which will depend on whether the affected nerve trunk is in a state of acute neuritis or quiet nerve paralysis. The actions to be taken in these cases are:

— refer the patient for confirmation of your diagnosis, detailed assessment of sensory loss and muscle weakness, and treatment;
— monitor and support the patient during the treatment programme.

Nerves in danger of destruction

- Record the degree of nerve involvement
- Refer the patient for:
  — confirmation of diagnosis
  — detailed assessment
  — treatment
- Monitor and support patient

Treatment of nerves in danger of destruction

Treatment of nerve trunks that have been damaged but not destroyed will have to be directed to the patient, to the affected nerve trunk and to the affected muscles and joints. Nerve trunks that have been destroyed (nerve involvement Grade 6) are not likely to recover with treatment.

Treatment of nerves in danger of destruction

- Treat patient
- Treat affected nerve
- Treat affected muscles and joints

Principles of treatment in acute neuritis

Patients with acute neuritis will require treatment for leprosy, and also for the complicating reactional state, erythema nodosum leprosum (ENL) or reversal reaction. They should therefore be referred without delay to persons competent to treat this condition.

The acutely inflamed nerve trunk will also need treatment to relieve the pain and reduce the inflammation, and to prevent internal strangulation of the nerve due to acute inflammation. When muscle weakness and deformity are present, the affected muscles and joints will also need treatment, to strengthen the muscles and to prevent the joints becoming stiff.

Principles of treatment in quiet nerve paralysis (QNP)

Patients with quiet nerve paralysis will require treatment for leprosy and also for the onset or worsening of nerve damage. They should be referred to a physician competent to treat this condition. Because the nerve trunk is not acutely inflamed, it will not require any treatment, such as splinting or heat, specifically directed to it. However, if muscle weakness is present, the affected joints and muscles will have to be treated, to prevent the joints becoming stiff and to strengthen the muscles.

The following table indicates the specific treatment that is required in these cases.

Target	Treatment	
	Acute neuritis	**Quiet nerve paralysis**

Patient	1. Anti-leprosy treatment
	2. In BL/LL cases[a] (ENL):[b]
	   — thalidomide[c]
	   — other anti-reaction
	    (ENL) drugs
	   — prednisolone
	3. In BB/BT/TT cases[d]
	   (reversal reaction):
	   prednisolone
		1. Anti-leprosy treatment
		2. Prednisolone

Affected nerve trunk	1. Rest (sling, splint, plaster cast) 2. Heat or ultrasound treatment of nerves 3. Surgery to relieve compression of nerves	No special treatment
Affected muscles	1. Active exercises 2. Electrical stimulation 3. Splints	1. Active exercises 2. Electrical stimulation 3. Splints
Affected joints	1. Massage 2. Assisted exercises 3. Splints	1. Massage 2. Assisted exercises 3. Splints

[a] BL refers to borderline lepromatous leprosy; LL refers to lepromatous leprosy.
[b] Erythema nodosum leprosum.
[c] Thalidomide should not be used in women of childbearing age. Such women should be given other anti-reaction drugs.
[d] BB refers to mid-borderline leprosy; BT and TT refer to borderline tuberculoid and polar tuberculoid leprosy, respectively.

Patients with acute neuritis or quiet nerve paralysis should be referred to the nearest medical facility where the above treatment is available.

What to do in acute neuritis

Acute neuritis of a nerve trunk is a serious condition, and if it is not treated, it may cause permanent damage to the nerve trunk within a few days. Patients with this condition should be referred immediately to an appropriate centre for treatment.

Acute neuritis

Refer patient immediately to an appropriate centre for treatment

---

There will be instances where the patient can get to the referral centre or clinic only after a few days, resulting in a delay in initiating treatment. In such situations, you should start treating the condition in order to avoid damage to the nerve trunk, and ensure that the patient goes to the treatment centre as soon as possible thereafter, in any case within 7–10 days. If the patient develops nerve paralysis during this period, however, he or she must go to the referral centre immediately.

Treatment at the field level is aimed at relieving pain and reducing inflammation. These aims are achieved by splinting the affected part, elevating it and giving the patient certain drugs.

Appropriate splinting of the affected part and keeping it elevated (see pages 42 and 78) will reduce inflammation and relieve pain to a considerable extent. However, the inflammation may be brought down rapidly by giving prednisolone (see below), if this is permitted. Permitting peripheral workers to initiate steroid therapy in cases of acute neuritis, when there would be some delay in getting the patient to the referral centre, is likely to help prevent nerve damage, and is unlikely to harm the patient. In addition, the patient may need medication for relief of pain. Acetylsalicylic acid (aspirin), which is also an anti-inflammatory drug, is probably most useful for this purpose. In most cases, a dose of 1000 mg three times a day will be sufficient.

Acute neuritis

In the case of a delay in the patient reaching the referral centre:

1. Initiate treatment:
   — splint and rest the affected part
   — start prednisolone therapy
2. See that the patient reaches the referral centre within 7–10 days

---

Prednisolone treatment under field conditions

It has been the practice to give treatment with prednisolone to only those patients under the supervision of a physician. This is because serious complications, e.g. high blood pressure, bleeding from the stomach and diabetes, may occur. Tuberculosis may also occur due to immunosuppression. However, some centres now permit prednisolone to be given by senior health workers, under field conditions, in order to make the benefits of the drug available to more patients.

For the purpose of preventing nerve damage, it is recommended to start treatment with a relatively high dose of the drug (40–60 mg per day) and change over to a lower maintenance dose of 30–40 mg per day, after two or three weeks. The maintenance dose should be given for at least three months, or until the drug is found to be no longer needed (patient fully recovered) or useful (no evidence of any recovery); then the dosage should be gradually reduced over 4–6 weeks before stopping it altogether.

Patients who receive prednisolone treatment should be checked frequently to ensure that:

— they are taking the drug as prescribed;
— they do not suddenly stop taking the drug;
— they are not developing complications.

If the patient is already known to have a chronic cough, frequent fever, chronic or frequent pain in the abdomen, high blood pressure or diabetes, you should bring that fact to the notice of the person prescribing the drug (physician or senior health worker). The physician or senior health worker should also be informed immediately if the patient develops any problem while under prednisolone treatment, even when the symptoms (e.g. cough, headache, swelling of ankles, abdominal discomfort, or septic infections) are apparently trivial and not troublesome. This is important, because a delay in recognizing complications resulting from prednisolone treatment may endanger the life of the patient.

Monitor patients during treatment

Patients with severe neuritis with or without severe reaction (ENL or reversal reaction) will need to be admitted to hospital and treated as inpatients. Those with quiet nerve paralysis or mild neuritis not requiring hospitalization will be examined and prescribed treatment and followed up as outpatients. Senior health care personnel will see these patients only periodically, the frequency depending on individual circumstances. Therefore, you will have to monitor these patients during the intervals between their visits to the clinic or hospital. The purposes of such monitoring are:

— to ensure that the patient is following the treatment advice (e.g. regarding taking the prescribed drugs, especially prednisolone, doing the exercises and wearing the splints, etc., as instructed);
— to verify whether the patient is improving;
— to assist the patient in carrying out the treatment advice where necessary;

— to ensure that the patient attends the clinic or hospital as advised;

— to check that no complications have arisen.

6.5 Instructing patients about preserving nerve function

Aims of instructions

As explained earlier, when a nerve trunk is thickened, it is not possible to predict at that stage whether it will become damaged and destroyed. This means that, apart from anti-leprosy treatment, there is little that can be done at that stage to protect the nerve and preserve its function. It is only when a nerve trunk starts getting damaged that it becomes evident that it is in danger of being destroyed, and measures can be initiated to prevent that happening. The earlier the nerve damage is recognized and treated, the better are the chances of recovery of that nerve. The patient therefore needs to be instructed about:

— the consequences of nerve damage;

— how to recognize the onset and worsening of nerve damage;

— the need for reporting signs of onset and worsening of nerve damage without delay;

— the possible preventive treatment that may be required.

Knowledge of consequences of nerve damage

For conveying information regarding nerve damage and its consequences, instruct the patients verbally and demonstrate the consequences. At least one other member of the patient's household should also be given this information and taught to assist the patient and participate in the patient's attempts at preserving nerve function.

Teach the patient and the family member that:

1. Nerve trunks supply areas of skin in the hands and feet and muscles in the hands, feet and eyes.
2. Nerve trunks can get damaged slowly and progressively, or suddenly.
3. When a nerve is damaged:
    — the affected area of skin does not sweat and becomes dry;
    — the affected skin loses its ability to feel pain, heat and touch;
    — the ability to feel pain and heat is lost earlier than the ability to feel touch;
    — abnormal sensations may occur in the affected area of skin;
    — certain muscles (of the hands, feet and eyes) become weak.

Recognizing onset and worsening of nerve damage

To recognize the onset or worsening of nerve damage, the patient must learn to look for:

— loss of sweating;
— changes in sensibility;
— muscle weakness.

The patient must learn:

- To check, by looking and feeling, whether there are any areas in the palms and soles that do not sweat and, if so, whether they are increasing in size.
- To notice any abnormal sensations (e.g. numbness or burning) confined to one area in the palms or soles.
- To check whether there is any loss of feeling of pain, heat or touch in any areas of skin in the palms and fingers (this must be done with care so that the palmar skin is not injured while testing it — detailed explanation as to how to do this should be given) and, if so, whether they are increasing in size.
- To check that all the fingers can open out fully and be kept together in that position; and that the thumbs can move freely in all directions.
- To check that the toes can be raised off the ground and held up for at least 30 seconds without drooping down; and that the feet can be held up for the same time without drooping.
- To check that the eyes are in good condition and the eyelids can close tight.

The patient, with the help of the family member, should carry out these checks systematically and regularly, e.g. once a month, and keep a record of the results. For this purpose, the patient should be provided with a checklist of what to look for. A sample checklist is given below.

Checklist of signs and symptoms of onset or worsening of nerve damage

1. Areas of non-sweating in palms and soles. Whether they are increasing in size.
2. Abnormal sensations in palms and soles. Their nature and location.
3. Ability to feel pain in palm and fingers.
4. Ability to feel heat in palm and fingers.
5. Ability to feel touch in palm and fingers.
6. Ability to keep fingers straight and together.
7. Ability to move thumbs all round.
8. Ability to raise toes off the ground.
9. Ability to keep feet lifted up.
10. Ability to close eyes tight.

Report without delay

The patient needs to be taught to report onset or worsening of nerve damage without delay. It must be explained that nerve damage can be arrested and the damaged nerve can recover if treated at an early stage, whereas later, recovery will not be possible as the nerve will have been destroyed. Patients should also be introduced to others who have benefited from early treatment, since this will reinforce the message.

Message

Nerve damage can be cured if recognized and treated early

Explain treatment

The patient must also be informed what kinds of treatment are usually given to arrest and cure nerve damage and why they are given, using simple language and familiar concepts. Patients must know:

— that they will need to take certain drugs as prescribed;
— that they may have to wear splints;
— that they may have to practise certain exercises and massage.

They should also understand the purpose of the treatment:

— to control the disease process;
— to rest the nerve so that it can recover faster;
— to keep muscles strong and joints supple.

Patients with acute neuritis should know that surgery may be required in order to make the drug treatment effective. The patients must be made to realize that efforts to preserve nerve function require their full cooperation with the health care personnel and that without this they will not succeed. In particular, patients must follow the instructions and treatment advice given. This is very important.

Message

- Preserving nerve function requires effort by the patient
- Drugs will control the disease process, if taken as prescribed
- Splinting will rest nerves and help their speedy recovery
- Exercise and massage will keep muscles strong and joints supple
- Sometimes surgery may be required

Summary

To arrest nerve damage and preserve nerve function:

— recognize nerve damage early;
— teach the patient to recognize and report the onset or worsening of nerve damage without delay;
— treat damaged nerves properly and adequately;
— encourage the patient to follow treatment advice.

CHAPTER 7

Instructing and training patients in disability prevention

7.1 Patient participation essential

Prevention of disabilities is a joint venture in which the patient has to participate fully as an equal partner. In order to prevent disability, the patient and the health care personnel must learn to recognize disability-prone situations and look for practices to avoid or prevent disability. In order to develop this kind of behaviour, the patient should know:

— what kinds of disabilities and deformities he or she may develop and how;
— that disabilities can be prevented by appropriate action;
— what those actions are and by whom they should be taken.

Patients should also be trained in practices appropriate to meet their requirements. This chapter discusses what patients should know and practise in the context of disability prevention.

Patients should know

- How disabilities develop
- How disabilities can be prevented by practices to preserve hands, feet, eyes and nerves

---

7.2 What patients should know about disabilities

Patients may not understand and may not be interested in the technical details of disabilities caused by leprosy. However, they should have a basic understanding of how these disabilities arise and what needs to be done to prevent them. They should know that:

- Leprosy can produce primary impairments involving the nerves, eyes and nose, that is, leprosy may directly damage these structures.

- Nerve damage gives rise to: loss of sweating and impaired sensibility over specific areas of skin of the palms and soles; weakness and paralysis of certain muscles in the hands and feet; and dryness and muscle weakness in the eyes.
- Insensitive and dry hands, feet and eyes get damaged easily and may be destroyed if injuries are neglected.
- Most of these consequences can be prevented by following certain practices.

Patients should also know which are the paralytic deformities that result from nerve damage and which are the anaesthetic deformities that result from neglected injuries. Thus, they should know that deformities such as claw finger, claw thumb, drop-wrist, drop-foot and lagophthalmos are paralytic deformities, since they are caused by damage to specific nerves and the consequent muscle paralysis.

Similarly, they should also know that other disabling conditions such as ulceration in the soles and palms, shortening of fingers and toes, stiffness of joints (also known as contractures) and mutilations are anaesthetic deformities, because they are caused by repeated, neglected injuries and wounds to insensitive hands and feet.

Message

1. Leprosy may damage the nerves, eyes and nose.
2. Nerve damage causes dryness, impaired sensibility and muscle weakness in the hands, feet and eyes.
3. Insensitive hands, feet and eyes get damaged and may be destroyed if injuries are neglected.
4. Damage to the hands, feet and eyes may be prevented by following certain practices.
5. Claw finger, claw thumb, drop-foot, drop-wrist and lagophthalmos are paralytic deformities.
6. Ulceration, shortening of digits, stiffness of joints and mutilations are anaesthetic deformities.

7.3 What patients should know about disability prevention

The patient should know that:

— disabilities and deformities can be prevented;
— he or she has to participate, as a partner, in the prevention programme;
— involvement of the nerves, eyes and nose (primary impairments) is prevented if leprosy is diagnosed early and treated with multidrug therapy;

— permanent damage to the nerve trunks and paralytic deformities can be avoided if nerve damage is recognized early and treated properly;

— paralytic deformities can be corrected by surgery;

— anaesthetic deformities are very difficult to correct by surgery or any other means, but can be prevented by practising hand care, foot care and eye care; and

— there are ways of protecting insensitive hands, feet and eyes and preserving nerve function.

7.4 What patients should do to preserve insensitive hands and feet

In order to preserve their insensitive hands and feet, patients should practise:

— general precautionary measures to prevent injuries and wounds;

— special care procedures to deal with specific problems such as dry skin, raw areas, deformity and swelling.

General precautionary measures

Insensitive skin does not feel pain, which is the signal of the body to let the person know that a part has been injured. Therefore, when an insensitive hand or foot is injured, the patient does not know and allows the injury to be repeated and worsen. In order to protect the insensitive hand or foot, the patient should know that an injury has occurred, review how it could have happened, work out a method of avoiding a similar injury in the future and take certain other general precautions.

The only way to find out whether an insensitive hand or foot has been injured is to examine it daily in good light for signs of injury, e.g. a wound, foreign body (piece of wood, metal or stone), blister, bruise, swelling or inflammation.

General precaution I

Examine hands and feet daily for evidence of injury

If an injury is noticed, the patient should review how the hand or foot was used and how the injury could have happened. The patient should then work out how a similar injury could be avoided in the future, i.e. what kind of protective measures he or she would have to take so that the same or a similar activity can be carried out safely, without causing injury.

> **General precaution II**
>
> Work out how the injury occurred and what protective measure will prevent it

Protecting hands

The patient should realize that any manual activity can injure an insensitive hand because no information reaches the brain about what is happening to the hand. Therefore, to protect the hand, the patient must take extra care, at home as well as at work, whenever the hand is being used. In order to do this, the patient must learn to think about the possibility of injuries occurring before starting to use the hand for any kind of activity. He or she must also learn to check the hand for injuries after every manual activity to ensure that it has not been harmed by that activity. The patient must learn to use any necessary protective aids or appliances such as mittens, gloves, towels or cloths, and modified tools with insulated handles, both at home and at work. The health worker should explain to the patient's family and workmates the reason for these precautions and enlist their support to encourage the patient to take all the necessary precautions. In any case, a patient with insensitive hands should check them each day for injuries.

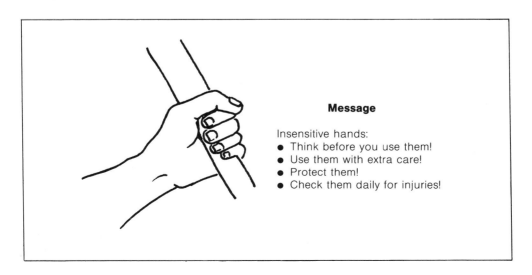

Message

Insensitive hands:
- Think before you use them!
- Use them with extra care!
- Protect them!
- Check them daily for injuries!

Protecting feet

The patient should know that:

- The main cause of disability in the insensitive foot is from persistent or repeated ulceration.
- Ulcers develop when the insensitive foot is injured and the injury is neglected because there is no pain.
- When an ulcer heals, a scar is formed. Walking causes the scar to break down and the ulcer to develop again.
- When ulcers occur in the sole, they become infected and that causes damage to the foot.
- The insensitive foot may be injured in two different ways: (i) by walking, which causes injury to the tissues under the skin in the sole, usually in the front part (ball) of the foot; and (ii) by external wounding due to contact with sharp or hot objects (Fig. 78).

Message

1. Main cause of disability in insensitive feet — ulceration.
2. Ulcers develop when injuries to insensitive feet are neglected.
3. Ulcers in insensitive feet recur when scars break down during walking.
4. Insensitive feet get damaged when ulcers in the sole become infected.
5. Insensitive feet may be injured by walking (internal injury) or by contact with sharp or hot objects (external wounding).

In short, the patient must become aware of the problem of insensitivity and its consequences so that he or she realizes the need for, and the kind of protective measures to protect feet from damage.

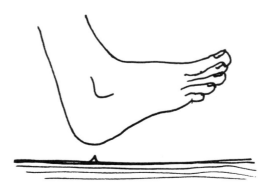

Fig. 78. External wounding of the foot

When the patient understands how and why ulcers occur, the protective measures are easily understood and are more likely to be complied with. In order to protect their insensitive feet from ulceration, patients must learn:

— to protect the feet from external injury;
— to protect the feet from walking strains;
— not to allow skin cracks to develop in the foot (see Fig. 79 and page 124).

Protecting insensitive feet from external injuries. Insensitive feet will be protected from external injury if the patient uses footwear that has a tough sole, resistant to penetration by thorns, etc. Rubber (from old tyres) is often used for the sole because it is tough and cheap. However, any hard or tough material may be used.

> Use footwear with a tough sole

The footwear must fit properly and be used correctly, with straps fastened as they should be. Buckles, if present, should not press on the insensitive skin and there should be no nails where they could injure the foot. In other words, the footwear should be safe and should protect the foot.

Protecting insensitive feet from walking strains. When the muscles of the leg and foot are weakened (see page 92), insensitive feet get damaged by the strains and stresses produced during walking. The damage occurs in the fatty tissue under the skin in the sole and can be avoided by reducing walking strains. Walking strains can be reduced in two ways: (i) by restricting walking to well within safe limits; and (ii) by using a suitable insole in the footwear.

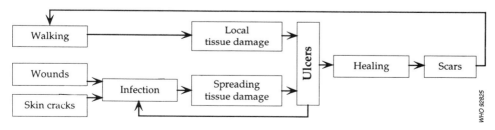

Fig. 79. Causes of ulcers in the foot

● *"Safe limit" for walking.* The patient should learn to recognize the safe limit for walking for his or her feet. After walking for some known distance (e.g. half, one or two kilometres), the patient should rest for about 20 minutes and then examine the feet systematically for signs of internal damage. These signs are:

— persistent warmth — the damaged part (usually the front part of the foot) feels warmer than the rest of the foot and warmer than the same part in the other foot;
— mild swelling or a blister some time later;
— a burning sensation or deep ache in one area;
— tenderness when pressure is applied to the same area.

If some or all of these signs are found, this indicates that the foot has been damaged and that the distance walked exceeded the safe limit for that foot. Fig. 80 shows where these signs are to be looked for in the front part of the foot. If no signs of internal damage appear, this indicates that the distance walked was within the safe limit for that foot. The patient will of course have to experiment for a few days to ascertain the safe limit for walking for his or her feet.

When the safe limit is exceeded

● Damaged part feels warmer and there may be mild swelling, a burning sensation or deep ache and tenderness
● Blisters may develop after some hours

If the patient has to walk distances much greater than the safe limit, the foot must be rested for 20–30 minutes before the safe limit is reached,

(a)   (b)

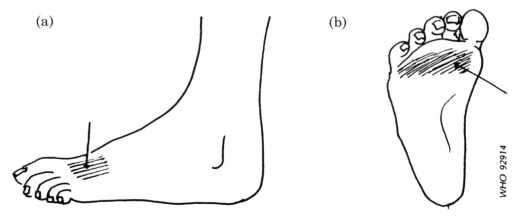

WHO 92914

Fig. 80. Sites of internal damage in the foot due to excessive walking

and then the journey resumed. It will of course be much better if such long or "unsafe" distances are not covered on foot at all, and some mode of transport is used instead.

Do not walk beyond "safe limit"

- Rest during prolonged walking
- Use some mode of transport for longer distances

- *Appropriate insole.* The simplest method to reduce strains during walking is to use footwear with a soft shock-absorbing cushion-like insole, which will reduce the pressure on the foot. Microcellular rubber or an equivalent synthetic substitute is generally used for this purpose. More specialized and custom-made footwear with moulded insoles will be needed for patients with badly scarred feet. The protective footwear must be used whenever the patient is standing or walking, inside the house as well as outside.

Reduce strains during walking by using footwear with a shock-absorbing insole
Use footwear all the time

The patient must also learn to take proper care of the footwear, keeping it in good repair and changing it as and when necessary.

Take care of your footwear

Explain to the patient the purpose of each part of the footwear (the tough sole for preventing external injury, the soft insole for reducing walking strains, etc.), so that he or she understands the importance of wearing the footwear to protect the feet and takes proper care of it.

Special care procedures

Special care procedures for specific problems

Besides the general precautionary measures, the patient will have to learn certain special care procedures, which will be needed to meet some specific problems. These problems are: (i) dry skin; (ii) skin cracks, wounds and ulcers; (iii) deformity; and (iv) swelling — all in the insensitive hands and feet. The procedures needed to deal with these problems are described in Chapters 4 and 5 and will not be repeated here. A brief summary of the principles underlying these procedures is given below. Health workers at all levels must ensure that patients become familiar with the procedures relevant to their individual needs.

Principles of skin care

Skin care procedures are necessary to overcome the problem of dryness and thickening of the skin (corns and callosities) in order to prevent skin cracks and ulcers. If dry skin is not cared for, it breaks, forming cracks and fissures, through which infection enters and spreads, extensively damaging deeper tissues of the hand or foot and leading to much disability.

Skin care procedures consist of:

— soaking the hand or foot in soapy or salty water;
— scraping the thickened skin;
— softening the skin with oil;
— when necessary, shaving the top layers of thickened skin.

These are described in detail on pages 39–40 and 58–59. Read them again and train the patients in these procedures.

Care of ulcers or raw areas

Practice of ulcer care procedures (including care of skin cracks and wounds) is necessary to get raw areas to heal as quickly as possible, which limits the damage to tissues and minimizes the amount of scar tissue. Essentially these procedures consist of:

— cleaning the raw area (ulcer, crack or wound);
— covering the raw area to keep it clean;
— resting the part and allowing it to heal.

These are described in detail on pages 30–37 and 66–70. Read them again and train the patients in these procedures.

Care of deformities

The leprosy patient may already have a deformity in the hand or foot. Disability prevention requires that this should not be allowed to become worse and complicated by the secondary impairment of stiffness of joints (contractures). In a deformity, some joints are held in a fixed position and some muscles may be weak. Care of deformities includes:

— care of joints to prevent stiffness or contractures which increase disability and make correction by surgery difficult;
— care of muscles to increase the strength of weak muscles.

The procedures include oil massage and exercises. These are described in detail on pages 45–49 and 73–74. Read them again and train the patients in the procedures of care of joints and muscles.

Care of the swollen hand or foot

The insensitive hand or foot may become swollen either because it has been injured or because it has become infected. If the swelling and its cause are not diagnosed and treated promptly, there will be extensive damage to the tissues of the hand or foot, which will cause severe disability. Therefore, it is most important to treat the swollen hand or foot with the greatest urgency. Essentially, you need to distinguish swelling caused by infection from that caused by injury to the deeper tissues, such as a bone or joint, and then treat the cause and the swelling. The management of swelling is described in detail on pages 40–43 and 75–79. Basically, it consists of elevation of the swollen part, rest to the part, and some kind of exercise. Read those pages again and train the patients in the initial management of swelling.

Care of nerves

Nerve care practices are meant to preserve the function of major nerve trunks by arresting nerve damage and promoting recovery of damaged nerves. These procedures are described in detail in the previous chapter. Read it again and train the patients in the care of nerves.

7.5 Instructing and training patients

Instruction and training

Instruction is communicating to the patient certain specific information — in this context about disabilities and how to prevent them. Training is helping the patient to become competent in carrying out the tasks necessary for preventing the onset or worsening of disabilities and deformities. While instruction is largely theoretical, training is highly practical. Instructions may be given through various channels, including discussions (formal and informal), books, audiovisual aids and demonstrations on volunteers (usually the most effective). Training is carried out by first demonstrating a task to patients and then letting them practise it under supervision until they can do it properly.

> **Instruction:** Informing the patient through discussions, books, audiovisual aids and demonstrations
> **Training:** Helping the patient to become competent in doing specific tasks

Purpose of instructing and training patients

Patients should be instructed and trained so that they can play their part in preventing disabilities, deformities and handicaps. Disability prevention cannot be a one-sided affair; it requires the two parties, health care personnel, and patients and their families, working together as partners for its success. Any amount of exercise, dressing of ulcers and the distribution of footwear and splints in clinics will not succeed in preventing disability if the patients remain only as passive recipients of services. Therefore, patients and their families must be instructed and trained in disability preventive behaviour to ensure their active participation in the programme.

> Instruct and train patients and their families to ensure their participation in the programme

Target persons

While it is obviously essential for the patient to be instructed and trained in disability prevention, it will make a lot of difference to the patient and to the success of the programme if at least one other member of his or her family (e.g. a parent or spouse) is also included in the instruction and training. This will also help to motivate and encourage the patient to practise disability prevention.

> Instruct and train a family member to support, help and encourage the patient

Community volunteers should also be instructed and trained in disability prevention. This will help to ensure that the patient is supported in his or her efforts by the community.

Some hints on instructing and training patients

There are no fixed rules about how to instruct and train patients in disability prevention. The methods will depend on local factors such as workload, competence of personnel and availability of resources. Nevertheless, the following general principles should be taken into account.

Keep it relevant

Whatever is taught should be seen by patients as relevant to their own problems. Otherwise they will have no interest in the information provided or in acting on it.

> Instruction and training should be relevant to patients' problems

Be intelligible

The purpose of instruction is to convey certain information to patients, so that they may act on the basis of that information, not to show how clever and well educated the instructor is. Therefore, the language and words used must be understandable to the patient. The message must be clear and unambiguous. This means that the instructor should avoid technical jargon and use simple and ordinary language instead. Similarly, the concepts and examples used must be familiar to the patient.

> Instruction should be intelligible
> Misunderstood information is unavailable information

Tackle one issue at a time

The instructor should resist the temptation to tell the patients everything that he or she knows about leprosy, disabilities, etc. If too much information is given, very little will be remembered. Whatever information is necessary and relevant should be given step by step, taking one problem or issue at a time, and moving on to the next one only after making sure that the patient has absorbed the information about the problem at hand and has become competent in the necessary practices and procedures needed for dealing with it.

> Avoid giving too much information
> Go step by step, taking one issue at a time

Help patients discover

People are always impressed by information and solutions they have discovered themselves. Information learnt in this way is remembered much better than information given by an instructor. Therefore, the instruction should be minimal, just sufficient to guide the patients. Let the patients talk and discuss by themselves and discover what has gone wrong, what problems that could lead to and how to avoid those problems. The instructor should function more like a signpost indicating the route to a given destination rather than a bus that carries the person to the destination. The instructor will learn a lot by listening to those who have learnt to live with problems. Group discussions involving patients with similar problems, their families and local community volunteers and discussions with individual patients will be very useful for instructing and training patients. Remember that instructing does not only involve talking to patients, but also listening to them and discussing with them.

> Let patients talk
> Listen and learn
> Help patients discover problems and solutions themselves

Be realistic

The purpose of disability prevention is to find practical solutions to patients' problems. The solutions that are offered or suggested must be feasible and practicable in the local context. Therefore, the instructor should be fully aware of the local resources regarding medical and surgical care, social welfare and rehabilitation, and confine solutions to what is feasible under local circumstances.

> Offer feasible and practicable solutions
> Be fully aware of local circumstances and resources

Be positive

It is easy to be pompous and tell patients that they should not do this or that. Many patients do not need such information (e.g. "don't touch hot things!") because they already know it. In any case, nobody likes being talked at in that manner. Instead, patients need to know what they should do. For example, it is meaningless to tell a patient with a plantar ulcer to avoid walking. What the patient should know is, given the condition of the foot, how he or she can get around safely. That will be more meaningful and is more likely to be acted upon than a command such as "don't walk!"

> Give positive instructions
> Tell patients what they should do, not just what they should not do

Have a planned instruction and training programme

Once the patients with disabilities and those at risk of disability have been identified in an area, a suitable disability prevention programme should be drawn up and implemented in stages. A planned programme of instruction and training, incorporating the available methods for preventing disability and structured to inform patients about their specific needs and train them in disability preventive behaviour, will be most desirable. It should also be flexible enough to meet individual needs.

> Have a planned instruction and training programme

Training patients to carry out specific tasks

In order to practise disability prevention, the patient will need to be trained to carry out certain specific tasks. These include the tasks involved in: protected use of hands at home and at work, protection of feet (see page 120), skin care, and care of ulcers or raw areas, deformities, swollen hands and feet, and care of eyes and nerves.

> **Train patients in**
>
> | | |
> |---|---|
> | Protected use of hands | Care of deformities |
> | Protection of hands | Care of swollen hands and feet |
> | Skin care | Care of eyes |
> | Care of ulcers | Care of nerves |

Remember that training in these procedures should be based on the needs of individual patients. Train a patient only in those tasks that are relevant to him or her. Demonstrate each step of each task, then ask the patient to do the same. The patient should practise the tasks until he or she can do them competently, without making any mistakes. Also periodically check, during monitoring visits, that the patient is doing the tasks correctly.

Train patients in relevant tasks only

- Demonstrate each task
- Make patients practise
- Correct wrong practices
- Ensure patients have been trained

The details of the various tasks have already been given in the previous chapters. Those relevant to training the patient are mentioned below.

Training in protected use of insensitive hands

Patients need to be trained to protect their insensitive hands from injuries at home and in the workplace. Such injuries usually occur during activities such as cooking, washing clothes and using tools with rough or sharp handles. Ask patients to demonstrate how they carry out these activities and show them how to avoid injuring their hands during these activities. When visiting patients, observe how they carry out the activities and correct any wrong and harmful practices. Where necessary, suggest that they use appliances or aids such as insulating handles on tools, or gloves, and help them to carry out your suggestions.

Protected use of insensitive hands

Train patients how to use insensitive hands without injuring them during activities such as cooking, washing and at work

---

Training in skin care

Patients need to be trained to take care of the dry insensitive skin of palms and soles and to prevent the development of cracks, by keeping the skin soft and supple. This is achieved by the daily practice of skin care. Therefore, teach patients how to soak their dry palms and soles and scrape the skin, either by rubbing the two palms (or soles) together or by using a scraper, and then soften the skin with oil.

> **Skin care**
>
> Train patients to soak insensitive hands and feet, and to scrape and soften the skin with oil

These procedures are described on pages 39–40 and 58–59. If you have any doubts, read them again.

Training in care of ulcers or raw areas

Ulcers need to be cleaned, dressed (at least every few days) and rested to heal. Clinics and hospitals will be unable to clean and dress ulcers as often as is necessary, and thus the patient (and preferably a family member) should be trained to clean the ulcer and surrounding area properly and keep the raw area covered or dressed using sticking plaster or gauze bandage.

> **Care of ulcers**
>
> Train patients how to clean and dress the ulcer

Show the patient and the family member how to wash and dry the ulcer and the area surrounding it. Also, demonstrate how to dress the ulcer, covering it properly with sticking plaster or gauze bandage. Observe how they carry out these procedures and correct any wrong practices. These procedures are described on pages 30–37 and 66–70. Read them again and refresh your memory so that *you* do not make mistakes.

Training in care of deformities

Patients with deformity of the hand or foot will need to be trained in care of the deformed part, in order to prevent crippling complications such as joint stiffness. For this purpose, the patient must practise oil massage and exercises.

> **Care of deformities**
>
> Train patients in oil massage and exercises

Show the patient how to apply oil and massage the hand and fingers or the foot and toes. Demonstrate the exercises for the hand or foot (whichever are relevant) to prevent joint stiffness and skin contractures. Observe carefully how the patient carries out these tasks and correct any wrong practices. These tasks are described on pages 45–49 and 73–74. Read them again and refresh your memory so that you can train the patient properly.

Training in care of the swollen hand or foot

Patients must be trained to recognize swelling of the foot (which is more common) and the hand at an early stage and take certain actions. The main action is to report the condition to you without delay. In the meantime the patient will also need to take certain other actions such as:

— resting the hand or foot in a sling or splint;
— applying a compression bandage;
— keeping the hand or foot raised above the level of the heart.

In any case, if the condition has not improved by these measures in 3–4 days, the patient must report to you.

Care of the swollen hand or foot

Train patients to recognize recent swelling,
to rest, bandage, and elevate the part, and
to report the condition without delay

These measures are described on pages 40–43 and 75–79. Read them again and refresh your memory as to how to deal with this problem.

Training in care of nerves

Patients must also learn to recognize the onset of nerve damage and its progress. For this purpose, the patient must learn to recognize any changes in sensibility in the hands and feet and the onset or worsening of muscle weakness. The patient and preferably one other family member must know how to assess the extent and nature of nerve damage, at least roughly. Therefore they should be trained to carry out simple methods of sensibility testing (for perception of pain, touch and, if feasible, heat) and to record the findings on a chart. These methods are described in the previous chapter. Read through it again so that you can train the patient properly.

> **Care of nerves**
>
> Train patients to test for impaired
> sensibility and record their findings on a chart

Periodically, or when felt necessary (e.g. when deterioration in the condition is suspected), the patient (and the other trained family member) should re-test and map the areas of impaired sensibility in the charts for comparison. They may also be trained to add other relevant information, e.g. the presence of claw deformity and muscle atrophy, to the charts. This will ensure that an objective record is kept of the patient's condition. It will also strengthen the patient's motivation to practise disability prevention.

Such training may also be given to groups of patients. In that case, they should keep each other's charts and compare the progress they have made among themselves. This will also strengthen their motivation to practise disability prevention.

CHAPTER 8

Monitoring and supporting patients

Monitoring refers to keeping a watch over patients to ensure that they are practising what they have learnt about disability prevention correctly. Supporting refers to providing and arranging for the necessary material, moral and social support to help patients practise disability prevention.

8.1 Importance of monitoring and supporting patients

It is not enough to instruct and train patients in disability prevention. If patients do not practise disability preventive measures properly, new disabilities will develop and existing disabilities will worsen. Therefore, for successful disability prevention, it is essential that instruction and training are followed up with monitoring and support.

> Monitoring and support are
> essential for ensuring success of
> disability prevention

8.2 Purpose of monitoring

The aims of monitoring patients are:

— to strengthen their motivation to practise disability prevention;
— to correct wrong practices;
— to detect new problems and solve them;
— to learn new solutions to problems.

To motivate patients to practise disability prevention

The patient will have to break certain old, harmful habits and develop new, protective ones in order to prevent worsening of existing disabilities and deformities and to prevent the occurrence of new impairments, disabilities and deformities. Breaking old habits and developing new ones requires the patient to make some extra effort, and may cause inconvenience and lead to additional expenditure. For these reasons, the patient needs to be encouraged to practise disability prevention and reminded about the importance of such practices for preventing the onset and worsening of disability. Monitoring also shows that you are serious about preventing disability and that you care about the patient's welfare.

To correct wrong practices

The patient may be practising what he or she has learnt about disability prevention, but may not be doing it correctly. By monitoring, you can identify any such wrong practices and help the patient to correct them. Monitoring is thus necessary to ensure that the patient practises disability prevention correctly.

To detect new problems

The patient may have developed new problems, impairments or disabilities, but may not be aware of them. By monitoring, you can detect any such problems, make the patient aware of them and help the patient to take the necessary actions.

To learn from patients

Many patients solve some of their problems on their own by clever and often inexpensive innovations. While monitoring, you can learn from such patients and apply similar solutions to others with similar problems.

8.3 Actions required

Monitoring requires three kinds of action on your part:

1. Assessing patients periodically for changes in impairment and disability status.
2. Talking with patients about their efforts at disability prevention.
3. Verifying patients' practices.

Assessment for monitoring

For monitoring purposes you need to assess and record the state of the patient's hands, feet, eyes and nerves periodically. This should be done regularly for the first two or three years and then once a year thereafter. Record the results in such a way that you can compare them with previous findings and identify any worsening of impairments and disabilities caused by the patient failing to practise disability preventive measures properly. Assessment for monitoring must be done regularly and systematically, and for this purpose it will be worth while carrying out these assessments on specific days and assigning this function to a specified person.

> Assess hands, feet, eyes and nerves regularly
> and systematically to identify worsening of
> impairments and disabilities caused by the patient
> failing to practise disability preventive measures

Verifying patients' practices

During visits to villages, or as part of a planned disability prevention programme, you should visit the patient's home (and workplace, if possible). The purpose of such visits is:

— to verify personally that the patient is practising disability preventive measures;
— to verify that the patient is carrying them out correctly.

During such visits, pay special attention to cooking and eating utensils, washing methods and work tools to ensure that they will protect and not harm the patient's insensitive hands. Also check that the patient is using proper footwear.

> Verify the patient's practices by visits
> Check washing methods, cooking utensils,
> tools and footwear

During your talks with the patient and visits to the patient's home and workplace, ask whether he or she has discovered any new ways of solving particular problems. You may be able to suggest similar solutions to others who have similar problems. Remember that even simple ideas may prove to be of major benefit.

> Learn from patients' experiences
> Communicate their ideas to others

Remember that the purpose of monitoring is to help patients practise disability prevention, not to find faults with them. At every stage, therefore, listen to patients and learn to appreciate their efforts and difficulties and make every effort to see how they may be resolved. Once you develop such an attitude, the difficult task of disability prevention becomes not only easier but also an interesting challenge.

> **Remember**
>
> Monitoring is not for finding faults
> It is for helping the patient to practise
> disability prevention

8.4 Supporting patients

Patients with permanent impairments and disabilities will need to practise disability prevention for the rest of their lives in order to prevent worsening of existing disabilities and the occurrence of new ones, especially those caused by unprotected use of insensitive hands and feet. The patient may need to use various aids, modified tools and other appliances at home and in the workplace, and do many things in a different way from others. Such "strange" behaviour may attract adverse comments, criticism or even frank disapproval from family members, neighbours and others. In such a hostile atmosphere, many patients find it difficult to practise disability prevention regularly, openly and properly. Therefore, the patient needs material, moral and social support from his or her family and others for regular, open and proper practice of disability preventive measures.

> **The patient requires**
>
> Material, moral and social support for
> regular, open and proper practice of
> disability prevention

Material support

Many patients require aids and appliances (such as protective footwear, gloves, splints, spectacles and modified tools with protective handles) to practise disability prevention. While some of these aids and appliances can be improvised, others must be made available to patients as part of the disability prevention programme. Even when the programme budget does not cover the costs of such aids and appliances, it is still possible to get them made locally or acquire them from elsewhere. If the patient cannot afford to pay for them, it may be possible to find a benefactor, such as a local service organization (e.g. a local benevolent group) who will be willing to cover the costs of supply. You should therefore identify the aids and appliances required for patients under your care and arrange for their supply from locally available services.

Aids and appliances

Identify requirements and arrange
for their supply

Such support, however small, will help the patient to practise disability prevention. However, remember that most people do not like to use aids and appliances, especially if that will make them appear conspicuous and different from others around them. Very often a simple, locally acceptable and inconspicuous modification is quite sufficient to serve the purpose and sophisticated appliances may not be needed at all. It is up to you and the patient and others interested in the patient's welfare to discover or improvise such modifications.

Aids and appliances must be
inconspicuous and acceptable

Having provided an appliance, whether it is protective footwear or a modified tool, you must verify that it is being used. If the patient is not using it, find out why and work out practical solutions to overcome the problem. Simply telling the patient to use it will not be effective.

Moral support

It is clear that the patient has to make extra efforts continuously and regularly to prevent the onset or worsening of disabilities and deformities.

The gains of disability prevention, after such efforts, are invisible and "negative" in the sense that only the consequences of failure are noticed, and when disability prevention has been successful there is nothing to be seen, since injuries, ulcers and stiffness, etc. are prevented. Under these circumstances, the patient may begin to lose interest in continuing with disability prevention. In order to prevent such weakening of motivation and to continue with disability preventive practices, the patient requires your encouragement and moral support. You must take an active interest in the patient's condition, give praise for his or her efforts at disability prevention, encourage the patient to continue and help the patient to solve any problems, when necessary, with positive and practicable suggestions.

Provide moral support:

- Praise the patient's efforts at disability prevention
- Encourage the patient to continue
- Give positive and practicable suggestions

Social support

As mentioned earlier, the patient practising disability prevention will, on many occasions, have to behave and do things in a different way from others, which may not be according to the locally established customs, practices and usage. This may lead to adverse comments, criticisms and even ridicule from family members, neighbours and others, which may discourage the patient from practising the necessary measures. For disability prevention to be successful, it is essential that the patient's family, co-workers, friends and others do not discourage the patient by their thoughtless comments and discriminatory behaviour. If the patient is supported in his or her efforts by family members and local society, practice of disability prevention becomes easy and successful.

Disability prevention by the patient requires support from family and local society

---

Such support will come only if the patient's family and others understand and appreciate why the patient needs to practise disability preventive measures and do certain things differently from others. This can be achieved by using formal means of health education such as audiovisual presentations as well as by informal means, such as group discussions in which patients also participate. During these discussions with family members, decision-makers (e.g. teachers and village elders) and targeted groups (e.g. students and women), patients express their difficulties and problems and the groups try to find some solutions. Discussion in groups is probably the most effective method for helping the patient's family and others to understand the problems involved in disability prevention.

> Make family members and others understand the
> patient's problems, difficulties and efforts
> by formal and informal means

By using these methods, you can convince the patient's family and others that the "strange" behaviour is necessary for protecting the patient from developing deformities and disabilities traditionally associated with leprosy and for preventing him or her from becoming severely disabled and a burden on others. You should be able to convince them that all societies accept and even prescribe non-customary behaviour and practices in certain circumstances. Maintenance of a person's health and preventing a person from becoming severely disabled is one such circumstance. When the patient's family and others realize this, you will find that they will not make the patient feel inferior or different and that they will actively encourage and support his or her efforts at disability prevention. Repeated discussions at individual and group levels may be required to bring about the required change in attitudes and behaviour of those concerned. Helping the development of such a positive and supportive attitude will go a long way towards abolishing the stigma associated with leprosy and leprosy-associated disabilities and deformities, enable leprosy patients and disabled persons to be accepted by society, prevent their dehabilitation and promote their rehabilitation within the local community.

> Convince people that non-customary behaviour
> and practices are necessary to maintain the
> patient's health and to prevent the patient from
> becoming severely disabled